JOHN A. BOSWICK, Jr., M.D.
University of Colorado Medical Center
Denver Colorado

emergency care

1981

W.B. Saunders Company

Philadelphia London Toronto Sydney

W. B. Saunders Company: West Washington Square
Philadelphia, PA   19105

1 St. Anne's Road
Eastbourne, East Sussex BN21 3UN, England

1 Goldthorne Avenue
Toronto, Ontario M8Z 5T9, Canada

9 Waltham Street
Artarmon, N.S.W. 2064, Australia

Library of Congress Cataloging in Publication Data

Boswick, John A., 1926–

Emergency care.

1. Medical emergencies — Handbooks, manuals, etc.
   2. Emergency medical personnel.   I. Title. [DNLM:
   1. Emergency medicine. WB 105 B747e]

RC86.7.B67   616'.025   81–50274

ISBN 0–7216–1876–6   AACR2

Emergency Care   ISBN   0-7216-1876-6

Last digit is the print number: 9   8   7   6   5   4   3   2   1

contributors

John A. Boswick, Jr., M.D., F.A.C.S.
Professor of Surgery, Chief, Hand Surgery Service, University of Colorado School of Medicine

William F. Bouzarth, M.D., F.A.C.S.
Professor of Neurosurgery, Medical College of Pennsylvania

Watson A. Bowes, Jr., M.D.
Professor of Obstetrics-Gynecology, University of Colorado School of Medicine

Henry C. Cleveland, M.D., F.A.C.S.
Clinical Professor of Surgery, University of Colorado School of Medicine

Robert J. Freeark, M.D., F.A.C.S.
Professor of Surgery, Loyola University School of Medicine

Robert W. Gillespie, M.D., F.A.C.S.
Associate Professor of Surgery, University of Nebraska College of Medicine

Oscar P. Hampton, M.D., F.A.C.S. (deceased)
Professor of Surgery (Emeritus), Washington University School of Medicine, St. Louis, Missouri

Larry Hatfield
Director, EMT Program, Lakeland Community College, Mentor, Ohio

Kenneth F. Kimball, M.D., F.A.C.S.
Clinical Assistant Professor of Surgery, University of Nebraska College of Medicine

Norman E. McSwain, Jr., M.D., F.A.C.S.
Professor of Surgery, Tulane University School of Medicine

James A. O'Neill, Jr., M.D., F.A.C.S.
Professor and Chairman, Division of Pediatric Surgery, Vanderbilt University Medical Center

Robert G. Osborne, M.D.
Associate Professor of Psychiatry, University of Nebraska College of Medicine

Mary Beth Skeleton, R.N.
Instructor in Surgery, Tulane University School of Medicine

William Vosik, M.D.
Clinical Assistant Professor of Internal Medicine, University of Nebraska College of Medicine

Robert F. Wilson, M.D., F.A.C.S.
Professor of Surgery, Director of Thoracic and Cardiovascular Surgery, Wayne State University School of Medicine

foreword

In the last several years in the United States, a variety of personnel delivering pre-hospital care has developed. There are two major standards, the EMT-A, who has completed the Department of Transportation Basic Ambulance Attendant Training Program, and the EMT-P, who has completed the National Standard Curriculum composed of 15 modules, developed under contract for the Department of Transportation. The curriculum has subsequently been accepted by most major medical organizations as well as the Departments of Labor and Health, Education, and Welfare.

This textbook has been developed as a companion to that training program. It can either be used within the training program to address some of the more common areas or be carried by the EMT as a handbook to refresh his knowledge between calls and to upgrade his skills.

For emergency department personnel, the chapter on extrication provides some insight into the environment that exists in the pre-hospital phase of care and the problems encountered by the EMT. It also helps explain to the emergency department personnel why the EMT does not immediately respond when asked to carry out a task in the field. The sterile environment present in the emergency department does not exist in the field, and, therefore, patient care is, in many instances, hampered by the less than ideal environment.

Because of the wide variety of personnel to which this text is aimed, there is variation in the scope of its chapters. It is hoped that this variation will assist the reader in his continuing quest for knowledge.

NORMAN E. McSWAIN, M.D.

preface

In 1964, *Emergency Care of the Sick and Injured* was prepared under the auspices of the Committee on Trauma of the American College of Surgeons. It was designed for law enforcement officers, fire fighters, ambulance personnel, rescue squads, nurses, and others involved in the first care of the sick and injured. The book was edited by the late Robert H. Kennedy and published by the W. B. Saunders Company. At the time of publication, paramedics, emergency medical technicians, nurse practitioners, emergency department specialists, and other emergency care personnel were unknown. This book was instrumental in the formation of training programs and courses in the field of trauma and emergency medicine. It was recognized as a galvanizing force in the improvement of the transportation and on-site and early care of the sick and injured in the United States.

In 1975, the Committee on Trauma of the American College of Surgeons voted to either revise this manual or publish a similar book. It was planned for the benefit of those who would render the first care to the sick and injured. The members of the Committee were aware that the first care for the sick and injured might be given by lay personnel, paramedics, emergency medical technicians, nurse practitioners, or emergency room doctors and nurses and recognized the difficulty in writing for such a diverse group.

The authors were chosen for their extensive experience in teaching or writing for the groups for which this book was intended. After several months of preparation, it was decided that it would not be appropriate for the Committee on Trauma of the American College of Surgeons to sponsor a publication for such a broad group. Many of those who had been asked to contribute to the book were convinced that there was a need for such a publication, however, and the editor and contributors decided to continue with the book. It was their feeling that this book should and would be read by a large number of paramedics, emergency medical technicians, ambulance drivers, emergency room nurses and physicians, and others interested in early emergency medical care. They felt that an updated publication of this type would be valuable to these groups and have designed this book for that purpose.

In preparing the final revision of each chapter, the editor and review committee have been extremely concerned with updating the material and presenting it in a manner that can be easily read and that is helpful to those who render the first or early care to the sick and injured.

The editor is deeply indebted to the late Dr. Oscar P. Hampton, Jr., who was active in the preparation of this publication until his death in December 1978. He had an opportunity to review the majority of chapters and offered suggestions that have made them appropriate for the intended audience.

JOHN A. BOSWICK, JR., M.D.

contents

CHAPTER

the emergency medical service system

The emergency medical service (EMS) system is a community's emergency response program for its citizens with injuries or illnesses needing urgent care. The system involves both pre- and in-hospital care. The pre-hospital phase begins when any citizen gives first aid or summons the emergency medical team. It continues with those providing rescue and emergency medical care at the scene and during transport to the hospital. The in-hospital phase includes care provided in the emergency department and definitive care.

A total EMS system should include the following:

Local and regional EMS councils
Public information and education
    Knowing what the system is and how and when
      to use it (information)
    First aid training, including CPR (education)
Detection and dispatch
The response system
    Vehicle
    Equipment
    Personnel

The emergency department
>   Appropriate back-up services (laboratory, radiology, ICU, and others)
>   Consultants and secondary hospitals
>   Rehabilitation
>   Evaluation and feedback into the system

Only some of these aspects are considered in this book.

PUBLIC INFORMATION AND EDUCATION

The public must know what the EMS system is and how to obtain access to it. They need to know the various ways in which help can be obtained. Stickers with the appropriate telephone numbers for emergencies are one way of providing public information.

Public education involves training the public as first responders. By requiring that all students have standard first aid before graduation from junior high school and advanced first aid before graduation from senior high school or before applying for a driver's license, we could ensure that within two generations almost everyone at the scene of an accident or an acute illness would be better able to save life and limb until professional help arrived.

THE AMBULANCE

The ambulance is an emergency response vehicle that has been developed to provide the working space and equipment needed to save patients' lives. Its design standards have been developed by the National Academy of Sciences and are mandated for vehicles purchased with federal funds. The Committee on Trauma, American College of Surgeons, has developed an equipment list describing the minimum support equipment that any ambulance should carry if it is providing emergency care (Table 1–1). Special requirements for the transportation of newborn infants are listed in Chapter 12.

All ambulances should be radio equipped for communication between the EMT-A and the physician in the emergency department. Ambulances staffed by trained EMT-Paramedics must have the capability of telemetry (vital sign transmission) to allow physician supervision and monitoring of EKGs.

Air ambulances are available in some areas for transport over long distances or difficult terrain. For basic emergency response, the essential equipment used in the ground ambulance should be carried. Access to the patient is required both while loading and during transport. The air ambulance used only for inter-hospital transfer should be equipped with those items needed to provide care for the patients being transported (not necessarily all the equipment on the equipment list).

TRAINING AND EDUCATION

The minimum level of training for the ambulance attendant should be that of the EMT-A or EMT-I (the 81-hour DOT course or its equivalent). Every ambulance should have at least two trained attendants at all times. EMT-As should have practical in-hospital experience during their training and, where possible, as part of their regular activity to maintain proficiency. They should meet on a regular basis with physicians and emergency department personnel to review problems and stay abreast of changes in patient care. Mistakes in care should be reviewed so that they can be corrected at once. Review sessions are better than infrequent refresher courses, although their frequency depends on the case load of the ambulance service.

EMT-Paramedics have advanced life-support training. They must successfully complete the standard federal EMT-Paramedic course and pass a certifying examination. Constant training is necessary to ensure that a high level of proficiency is maintained. Review sessions are preferred over annual refresher courses.

Emergency department personnel should be educated to the RN level. Regular continuing education must

Table 1–1   EQUIPMENT FOR AMBULANCES*

Essential†
Portable suction apparatus with wide-bore tubing and rigid
   pharyngeal suction tip
Hand-operated bag-mask ventilation unit, with adult, child, and
   infant size masks (clear masks are preferable); valves must
   operate in cold weather, and the unit must be capable of use with
   an oxygen supply
Oropharyngeal airways in adult, child, and infant sizes
Mouth-to-mouth artificial ventilation airways for adults and children
Portable oxygen equipment with adequate tubing and semi-open,
   valveless, transparent masks in adult, child, and infant sizes
Mouth gags, either commercial or those made of three tongue
   blades taped together and padded
Universal dressings, approximately 10 in × 36 in, compactly folded
   and packaged in convenient size
Sterile gauze pads, 4 in × 4 in
Soft-roller self-adhering bandages, 6 in × 5 yd
Roll of aluminum foil, 18 in × 25 ft, sterilized and wrapped
Two rolls of plain adhesive tape, 3 in wide
Two sterile burn sheets
Hinged half-ring lower-extremity traction splint (ring 9 in in
   diameter, overall length of splint 43 in) with commercial limb-
   support slings, padded ankle hitch, and traction strap
Uncomplicated inflatable splints
Short and long spine boards with accessories
Triangular bandages
Large size safety pins
Shears for bandages
p. 131 Sterile **obstetrical kit:** gloves, scissors, umbilical cord clamps or
   tapes, sterile dressings, towels, and plastic bags; burn sheets may
   be used as drapes if necessary
Poison kit: syrup of ipecac and activated charcoal
Blood pressure manometer, cuff, and stethoscope
Compartmentalized pneumatic trousers with inflation equipment
Two-way radio allowing direct communication between EMT and
   emergency department at hospital
Additional‡
Tracheal intubation kit
Pleural decompression set

Table 1–1 EQUIPMENT FOR AMBULANCES *(Continued)*

Drug injection kit
Venous cutdown kit
Minor surgery kit
Tracheostomy or cricothyrotomy set
Urinary catheters
Portable cardioscope and defibrillator
Access and Extrication§
Triangular reflectors or battery-operated flares
Wrench, 12 in long, with adjustable open end
Screwdriver, 12 in long, with regular blade
Screwdriver, 12 in long, Phillips type
Hacksaw with 12-in wire (carbide) blades
Pliers, 10 in long, vise-grip
5-lb hammer with 15-in handle ⎫
Fire axe butt with 24-in handle ⎬ (can be either separate or
24-in wrecking bar ⎭ combined as forcible entry tool)

Crowbar, 51 in long, with pinch point
Bolt cutter with 1¼-in jaw opening
Portable power pack (Portapower) and spreader tool
Shovel, 49 in long, with pointed blade
Double-action tin snip at least 8 in long
Two manila ropes, each 50 ft long and 3/4 in in diameter
Hard hat
Safety goggles

---

*From the Bulletin of the American College of Surgeons, May 1970; revised June 1975 and September 1977.

†Litters and safety and housekeeping equipment are not specified, since it is assumed that these basic items, as well as installed suction and oxygen, will always be carried.

‡May be carried in a sealed container, depending on local conditions and decisions (for use by EMT-Intermediate and EMT-Paramedic).

§Unless a rescue vehicle accompanies an ambulance on every accident call.

Note: A heavy-duty (2-ton) Come-along is recommended, particularly in areas where it would not otherwise be readily available. In addition to rated cable, the ambulance should carry a 15-ft rated chain with one grab hook and one running hook.

be provided, and in-hospital rotation will prove valuable in those institutions where the emergency department load is light. Standing orders and treatment protocols are established by the medical staff.

HOSPITAL RESOURCES

Not every hospital is properly equipped to care for seriously injured or critically ill patients. The American College of Surgeons is currently revising its suggested criteria for the designation of a hospital as a Trauma Center. Similar suggested minimums for other areas of care should be forthcoming.

The location of referral hospitals where optimal resources are available must be known to emergency departments and physicians. The decision to refer a patient is made only by a physician. (It is possible that local physicians will have established standing orders for the assignment of certain types of emergency patients to specific facilities.)

primary assessment of the critically ill and injured

Time is a crucial factor in managing emergency situations. It is essential that treatment follow an order appropriate to the direness of the conditions present.

Primary assessment of an emergency patient involves the functions of respiration and circulation, consciousness, and the possibility of injury to the cervical spine and consists of the following steps, in sequence:

1. Evaluate **airway** — restore open airway if needed and ensure its continued patency.

2. Ensure effective respiratory exchange — seal open wounds of chest, temporarily immobilize flail segments, and perform thoracocentesis or tube thoracostomy when needed.

3. Restore circulation by cardiopulmonary resuscitation when necessary. Maintain effective circulation by giving lactated Ringer's solution through a large-bore intravenous line. If travel time to the emergency department will exceed two hours, insert an indwelling urinary catheter.

p. 11

4. Cover open wounds, using pressure to control bleeding where necessary.

5. Perform a rapid but complete physical examination avoiding excessive movement of the patient, especially if spinal injury is suspected.

6. Start a flow sheet to record important observations: level of consciousness, pupil size and reactivity, and vital signs.

7. Obtain history of injury and events prior to and following the accident. Inquire as to allergies, medications, past illnesses, and last meal.

8. Before moving the patient, splint obvious or suspected fractures and the cervical spine in patients with head injuries. Examine for vascular and nerve injuries and record findings.

9. Notify the emergency department when immediate special examinations are indicated such as laboratory tests or radiographic examination.

In the initial assessment of an injured patient, it is often helpful to consider the human body as consisting of three regions. The *head and neck region,* which includes the brain and spinal cord, frequently sustains the most lethal injuries. Unfortunately, such injuries often lead to death irrespective of the quality of emergency medical care.

The *torso region* includes the chest and abdomen and is also commonly involved in life-endangering injuries. Early diagnosis and prompt treatment in this region will greatly affect the patient's chances for survival, but the facilities of a modern hospital are usually equally important.

The *extremities region* includes the shoulders, arm, forearm, and hand as well as the hip, thigh, leg, and foot. Injuries to these sites are rarely life endangering. They are, however, everyday occurrences and therefore are the principal cause of temporary or permanent disability. One has only to contemplate what the loss of function of even one finger might mean to an accomplished musician or the loss of a leg to a young dancer to appreciate the need for optimal care. Moreover, multiple extremity fractures with open wounds can produce shock, requiring prompt treatment.

General principles that should guide conduct during primary assessment include the following:

1. Avoid moving the patient unnecessarily.

2. One person should take charge of the patient.

3. Except for life-threatening problems, do not initiate treatment of obvious injuries (e.g., covering wounds) until evaluation of the patient is completed.

4. A satisfactory response to fluid replacement is apparent when pulse rate decreases, arterial blood pressure increases, skin color and temperature improve, and urinary output exceeds 30 ml per hour.

Persons attending women of childbearing age in emergency situations should keep in mind that the patient might be pregnant.

respiratory emergencies

Breathing consists of inspiration and expiration. Inspiration expands the chest, decreasing pressure within the alveoli of the lungs so that atmospheric pressure can force air in. Expiration compresses the alveoli to force air out.

The lungs are separated from the thoracic cage by the pleural space. The visceral pleura lines the lung side of this potential space, and the parietal pleura lines the thoracic cage side. During inspiration the diaphragm and intercostal muscles contract, expanding the thoracic cavity downward and laterally. Because the pleural space is only a potential space, the lungs expand into it. Decreased (negative) pressure is produced in the alveoli, causing them to be filled with air.

For effective exchange of oxygen and carbon dioxide, the air entering the lungs must be brought into close contact with the blood. The alveoli are lined with thin-walled capillaries, allowing this proximity. Any pathological process that causes a breakdown of the alveoli and their enlargement into the air sacs significantly decreases gaseous exchange by decreasing surface area.

Look at the nares to see if they are opening and relaxing. Watch the chest for normal and symmetrical expansion. Look for retraction of the suprasternal, supraclavicular, or intercostal areas, indicating an obstruction. Look for paradoxical movement of any part of the chest and for an open wound into the thoracic cavity. Observe the abdomen for movement, indicating that the diaphragm is working.

Listen with the ear to the mouth to reaffirm that there is good movement of air out of the nose and mouth. With the stethoscope, listen to the chest anteriorly and posteriorly. Pay particular attention to the upper part of the chest on each side. Normal breath sounds should be equal on both sides. Abnormal breath sounds are wheezes (whistling), moist rales (bubbling), or rhonchi (rattling).

Feel for air movement from the nose and mouth. Feel the entire thorax for areas producing pain, suggesting a fractured rib or a loose segment. Feel for wounds or lacerations. Feel for abnormal movement of the chest wall. Feel for paradoxical movements.

OBTAINING AND MAINTAINING A PATENT AIRWAY

Open the mouth and clear it of blood, mucus, vomitus, or foreign bodies. If a suction device is not at hand, the area may be cleared with a finger. If the patient is not breathing, start artificial ventilation (CPR) immediately. If he is trying to breathe but is moving little or no air, there is obstruction below the pharynx.

If there is no trauma and the respiratory arrest appears to be due to medical conditions, open the airway by hyperextending the head (Fig. 3–1). Place one hand on the forehead and the other behind the occiput (back of the head) or under the chin and tilt the head backward. This brings the oropharynx posteriorly away from the tongue. Air can then pass around the tongue and into the larynx. This is one of the most effective methods of

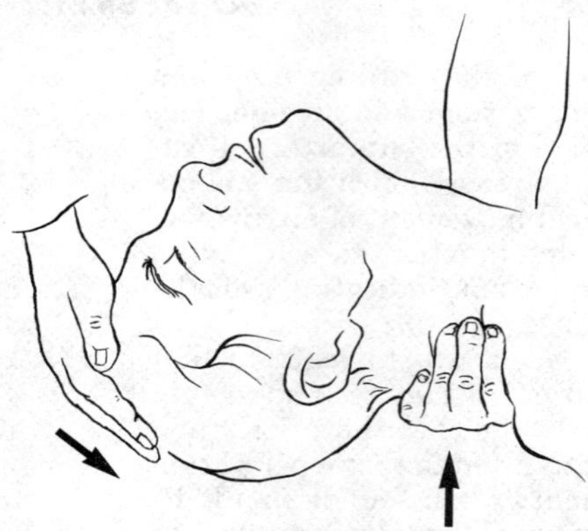

Figure 3–1 Opening the airway posteriorly.

opening the airway in patients without trauma. In an
unconscious patient with trauma, the airway should not
be opened in this manner because it can aggravate
cervical spine injuries. The possibility of cervical fracture exists in any patient with trauma to the clavicles
and upward or if the trauma patient is unconscious.

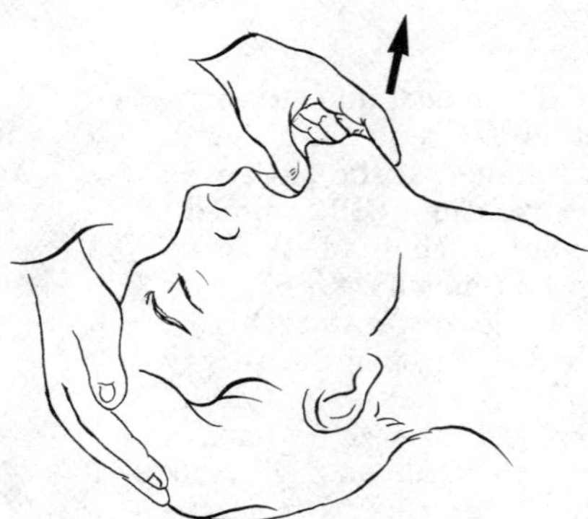

Figure 3–2 Opening the airway
anteriorly.

The airway can also be opened by lifting the mandible and tongue forward as a unit. This is the best method when the possibility of cervical spine fracture exists. Grasp the lower teeth and pull the mandible forward (Fig. 3–2). An alternative and more effective method is to place the long fingers behind the angle of the mandible on both sides and the thumbs on the cheek bones. The pressure of the long fingers juts the jaw forward. This is called the jaw jut maneuver.

Foreign Bodies

The upper airway may be occluded by a foreign object such as a piece of meat trapped in the larynx superior to the vocal cords. The patient is obviously choking and will turn cyanotic, particularly in the face and neck. There frequently is no loss of the ability to exhale. Therefore, the lungs become completely evacuated except for air that remains as dead space.

Because early recognition of airway obstruction is the key to successful management, it is important to differentiate this emergency from fainting, stroke, heart attack, epilepsy, drug overdose, or other conditions that cause sudden respiratory failure. Either partial or complete airway obstruction may be caused by foreign bodies. In partial airway obstruction the patient may dislodge the particle by coughing if there is good air exchange. If there is poor air exchange the signs will be a weak ineffective cough, high-pitched noises while inhaling, increased respiratory difficulty, and possible cyanosis. With complete airway obstruction the patient is unable to speak, breathe, or cough. He may clutch his neck.

Three manual maneuvers are used for relieving foreign body obstruction. They are back blows, manual thrust, and finger probe.

Back blows are a rapid series of four sharp blows delivered with the heel of the hand over the spine and between the shoulder blades. They may be administered with the patient sitting, standing, or lying and should be applied forcefully in rapid succession. Whenever possible, the patient's head should be lower than his chest to make use of the effect of gravity.

The child who has partial airway obstruction (is moving some air) should not be turned upside down because this may impact the foreign body against the undersurface of the vocal cords, resulting in complete obstruction. The child should be turned upside down only if he has complete airway obstruction. In this case, the obstruction cannot be made more serious, and turning the child upside down may possibly help.

Manual thrust, or the **Heimlich maneuver,** is a rapid series of four thrusts to the upper abdomen or lower chest that forces air out of the lungs to dislodge the foreign object (Fig. 3–3*A,B*). The **abdominal thrust** may be performed with the patient standing, sitting, or lying (Fig. 3–3*C*).

If the patient is standing or sitting, the rescuer should stand behind him and wrap his arms around the patient's waist. Place the thumb side of one fist high against the patient's abdomen and cover it with the open palm of the other hand. Then pull backward and upward in four rapid and forceful thrusts.

If the patient is supine, the rescuer may be either astride or alongside him. Turn the patient's head to one side. Place the heel of one hand against the patient's abdomen between the xiphoid process and the navel. Place the other hand on top of the first. Give a quick upward thrust into the abdomen.

The **chest thrust** is an alternate technique that is particularly useful when the abdomen of the patient is so large that the rescuer cannot fully wrap his arms around it or when pressure applied directly to the abdomen is likely to cause complications, as in advanced pregnancy. If the patient is standing or sitting, reach around from behind, placing your arms directly under the patient's armpits and around the patient's chest. Make a fist and place the thumb side on the breast bone but not on the xiphoid process or on the margins of the rib cage. Grasp this fist with the other hand and exert four quick backward thrusts.

If the patient cannot sit or stand, he should be placed on his back with his head turned to one side. The hand

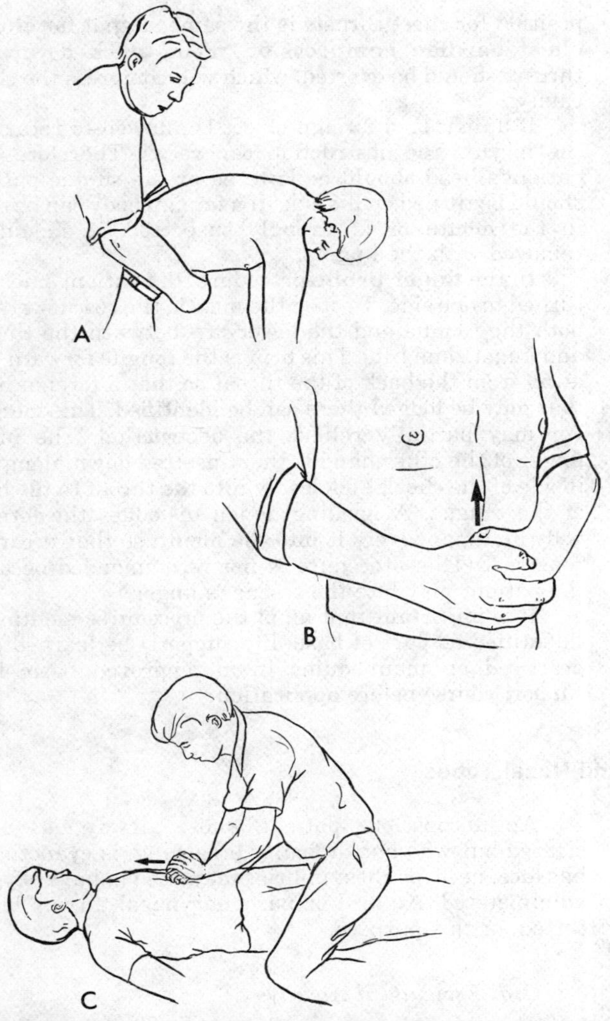

Figure 3–3 *A* and *B*, The Heimlich maneuver. *C*, The abdominal thrust.

position for chest thrusts is the same as that for **closed chest cardiac compression**. Four quick downward thrusts should be exerted, which will compress the chest cavity.

If a dislodged foreign object is allowed to return to the larynx, the obstruction can recur. Therefore, the patient's head should be lowered or the supine patient should be turned on his side. If a foreign body can be seen in the mouth or is strongly suspected, it should be removed with the fingers.

In the **finger probe** procedure, the patient's head is turned to one side. To open the mouth, the rescuer grasps both the tongue and the lower jaw between the thumb and fingers and lifts. This brings the tongue forward and away from the back of the throat so that a foreign body that may be lodged there can be identified. This maneuver may partially relieve the obstruction. The index finger of the other hand is then inserted down along the inside of the cheek and deeply into the throat to the base of the tongue. A hooking action dislodges the foreign body and maneuvers it into the mouth so that it can be removed. (This procedure is not recommended because the patient may bite the rescuer's finger.)

It is important that all of the procedures mentioned (identified as part of basic life support) be learned and practiced on mannequins in an approved basic life-support course before application.

Oral and Nasal Tubes

An unconscious patient whose airway has been cleared but who has difficulty breathing, is cyanotic, or has face, neck, or chest injuries may need to have oxygen administered. An oral or nasopharyngeal airway is inserted for this purpose.

Oral Esophageal Airways

An oral airway is an effective mechanical means of maintaining the tongue anteriorly to prevent blockage of the hypopharynx. The oral airway is a gently curving plastic or metal device that follows the anatomy of the oropharynx and hypopharynx. It rests on top of the tongue, below the hard and soft palates and anterior to the mucous membrane lining of the hypopharynx.

It must be emphasized that any object that touches or rests on the soft palate will produce wretching, gagging, or vomiting in a conscious patient. Care must be taken to assure that this gag reflex is not intact. Any vomiting at this stage most probably will result in aspiration and the difficult pneumonitis that surrounds this chemical inflammation of the alveoli and bronchus.

There are two mechanisms for the insertion of an oral airway. One is to insert the airway with the concavity directed cephalad until the soft palate is reached. At this point it is rotated with the concavity directed downward so that it follows the top of the tongue until it is secured into position.

The second mechanism utilizes some mechanical means, such as a tongue blade, to bring the tongue forward and slip in the oral airway with the concavity directed downward into its proper position.

Oral airways have the particular advantage of allowing a large tonsil suction device to be placed on either side and into the hypopharynx, providing an access for the removal of foreign material.

Nasopharyngeal Airways

A nasal airway is a soft, round tube that conforms to the anatomy of the nares, nasopharynx, and hypopharynx. It is inserted through either one or both nares to come to rest with the opening just above the epiglottis. The nasal airway has the advantage of being able to be frequently inserted in a patient whose gag reflex is still intact without producing vomiting. It has the disadvantage of being of such a small size that only a flexible suction tube will fit through it. It will not allow a larger tonsil suction to pass. Before inserting a nasal airway, lubricate the outside of the tube. Then pass it gently through the nose until the flange at the hilt is against the nose.

Esophageal Obturator Airway

The esophageal obturator airway (EOA) is one of two devices designed to isolate the trachea from the esophagus. It has several advantages: (1) it can be placed with the patient's head in the neutral position; (2) it can be placed rapidly, usually within 10 seconds; and (3) it does not require the use of a laryngoscope. The insertion procedure for this airway can be more easily learned, and the skills are retained much longer than those for insertion of the more complicated endotracheal tube. The complications of using this airway, which must be anticipated and avoided, include inappropriate placement in the trachea and vigorous insertion into the esophagus, which could cause perforation of the hypopharynx. The latter complication can be avoided by using a simple, gentle technique. The former can be avoided by listening with the stethoscope to both lungs for the presence of breath sounds after insertion of the airway and listening over the stomach to assure that air is not moving through the esophagus into the stomach.

The EOA functions just like an oral esophageal airway in that the tongue is held forward to allow passage of air into the trachea. The face mask seal must be as adequately maintained as when utilizing the bag valve mask with the oral airway.

Inflation of the esophageal balloon prevents regurgitation of gastric contents into the hypopharynx or its aspiration into the lungs as well as distention of the stomach by air proceeding down the esophagus.

The esophageal obturator is inserted by utilizing the jaw lift method to raise the mandible and the tongue anteriorly while maintaining the head in a neutral position. The well-lubricated EOA is then inserted gently into the esophagus to the full length of the tube. The balloon is gently inflated, the bag is squeezed while listening to the lungs to ascertain that it is in the proper position, and then the full 35 cc of air is placed in the esophageal balloon.

Ventilation is continued while maintaining a tight face mask seal. Although somewhat harder to ventilate than the bag valve mask and oral airway, the esophageal airway provides an adequate means of isolating the esophagus from the trachea in an emergency situation in which there is a possibility of cervical spine injury.

The esophageal gastric tube airway (EGTA) is a variation of the EOA. It allows a nasogastric tube to be placed down the center of the device to relieve pressure build-up in the stomach. This should reduce wretching and excessive pressure on the distal esophagus, which is occluded by the balloon.

Endotracheal Tube

The endotracheal tube is the ideal device, in many situations, for assuring an adequate airway. The tight face mask seal is not required. The trachea is well separated from the esophagus. It has the disadvantage of requiring skill and experience in insertion, and it is usually contraindicated in a cervical spine fracture.

The endotracheal tube is inserted by first sufficiently oxygenating the patient by hyperventilation. The head is placed in the "sniffing" position, with the neck flexed forward and the head extended back. The bag valve mask and oral airway used for hyperventilation are removed. The laryngoscope is inserted on the right side of the patient's mouth, moving the tongue to the left and visualizing the cord by lifting on the laryngoscope (not pivoting on the teeth). If a straight blade is utilized, the epiglottis is elevated with the tip of a blade. If a curved Macintosh blade is utilized, the epiglottis is elevated by placing the tip of the blade in the vallecula.

After the cords have been well visualized, the endotracheal tube should be inserted (Fig. 3–4). Appropriate positioning of the endotracheal tube is assured by listening over both lungs and the stomach with a stethoscope. The patient who is hypoxic initially, even if hyperventilated, may not have the adequate respiratory reserve to tolerate prolonged attempts at intubation. The astute operator should begin to count seconds when the bag valve mask is first removed from the patient. If, when a count of 15 is reached, intubation has not been ac-

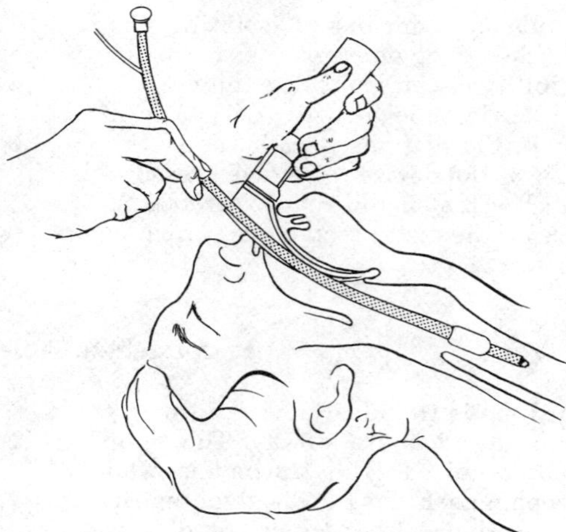

Figure 3–4 Establishing an airway by endotracheal intubation.

complished, further attempts should be stopped and bag
valve mask ventilation continued to resupply the patient
with oxygen. When he has been hyperventilated again,
further attempts at intubation can be continued.

Surgical Openings of the Airway

These are surgical procedures and should be em-
ployed only by trained personnel and only in extreme
emergencies.

Cricothyroid puncture consists of the insertion into
the trachea of a 13- or 14-gauge needle attached to a
syringe. The fingers of one hand are used to immobilize
the thyroid cartilage, and the notch beneath the thyroid
and above the cricoid cartilage is palpated with the other
hand. The needle is inserted through the skin, fascia,
and cricothyroid membrane. Continuous negative pressure is applied to the syringe until air is freely returned,
and the syringe is then removed.

Cricothyroidotomy is an incision in the skin, fascia, and cricothyroid membrane made to allow insertion of a tube in the trachea. The trachea is held with one hand, and the incision is made transversely.

ARTIFICIAL VENTILATION

Mouth-to-Mouth Technique

After the airway is opened by the jaw lift or jaw thrust maneuver and, if available, an oral airway is inserted, begin mouth-to-mouth ventilation, with the force and duration of each breath gauged by the size of the patient and the effectiveness of chest expansion. In infants, mouth-to-nose ventilation may be more successful.

Twelve breaths per minute are adequate for an adult. The respiratory rate should be about 20 to 40 breaths per minute for children under two years of age and 15 to 25 breaths per minute for children aged two to six. Auscultation of the chest is essential to make certain that both lungs are ventilated adequately.

Bag-Mask Resuscitation

A properly sized mask and self-inflating bag, when available, are much more efficient means of artificial ventilation if the airway is patent. Supplemental oxygen is advantageous. If respiratory exchange is still inadequate, endotracheal or EOA intubation is necessary.

Preventing Aspiration

Trauma is frequently accompanied by paralysis of the GI tract and gastric distention. The patient also may have eaten just prior to being injured. Such circumstances greatly increase the tendency to vomit, with aspiration of gastric contents. The stomach should be emptied as soon as possible using suction and nasogastric tube, and continuous suction should be maintained. If a nasogastric tube is not available, the patient should be positioned on his side so that aspiration is less likely.

p. 81 If there is any possibility of **spinal injury,** the back and neck must be kept immobile.

MANAGEMENT OF CHEST WOUNDS

Sucking Chest Wounds

When there is an open chest wound air will be sucked through the chest inspiration. When the thoracic cage contracts on expiration, air is expelled. Insufficient air will follow the normal pathways of the nose, mouth, nasopharynx, larynx, and trachea to allow adequate ventilation and expansion of the lungs.

Sucking chest wounds must be closed promptly. Place a nonporous material, such as Vaseline gauze, cellophane, or Saran Wrap, over the wound. Taping a square of cellophane on three sides and leaving one side open will allow air to be expelled but not sucked in. Such an arrangement tends to prevent **tension** p. 24 **pneumothorax.**

Flail Chest (Figure 3–5)

A flail chest is produced when two or more adjacent ribs are fractured in two or more places. If the fractures are on both sides there will be greater stability of the chest wall and less compromise of ventilation than if they were on the same side. If a segment of the thoracic cage is free floating, it will be pushed in by normal atmospheric pressure, decreasing the ability of the lungs to expand on inspiration. On expiration, increasing pulmonary pressure should force air out of the lungs, but the segment that has lost its integrity will bulge outward so that the ability of the thoracic cage to force air out of the lungs is decreased. This to-and-fro motion of the flail segment (so-called paradoxical respiration) pre-

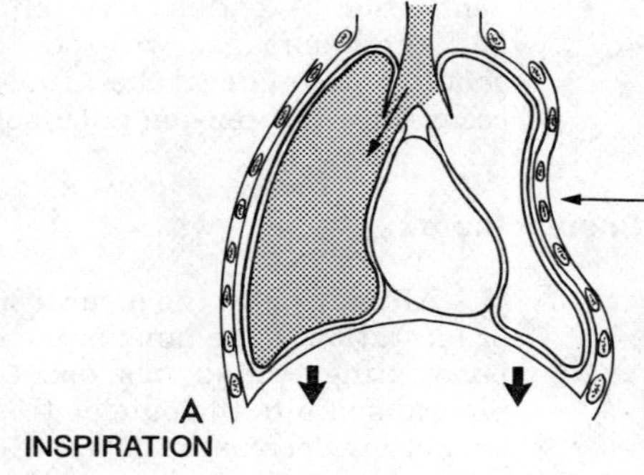

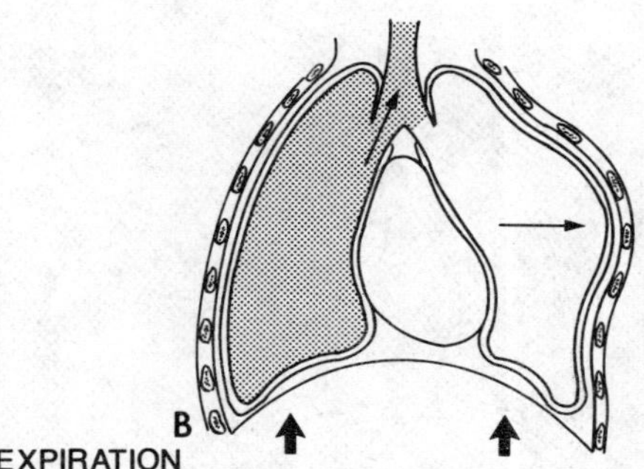

Figure 3–5 Flail chest. The chest wall on the affected side moves inward on inspiration and outward on expiration.

vents adequate ventilation. The movable segment of the thoracic cage must be stabilized so that paradoxical movement is eliminated.

External stabilization is accomplished by taping a pillow, a rolled shirt, or an IV bag over the loose segment so that it is held in. Outward movement should then be impossible. The straps from the short backboard can also be used to maintain the pillow in position.

Internal stabilization is accomplished by inserting an endotracheal tube and providing positive pressure ventilation. A patient with blunt thoracic trauma and flail chest managed with positive pressure ventilation should have bilateral chest tubes inserted to prevent the occurrence of a tension pneumothorax.

Pneumothorax

Air may enter the pleural space when there is a tear or laceration of the lung, bronchus, or trachea or when a penetrating wound has opened a pathway from the pleural space to the outside (Fig. 3–6A). The accumulation of air decreases the area into which the lungs can

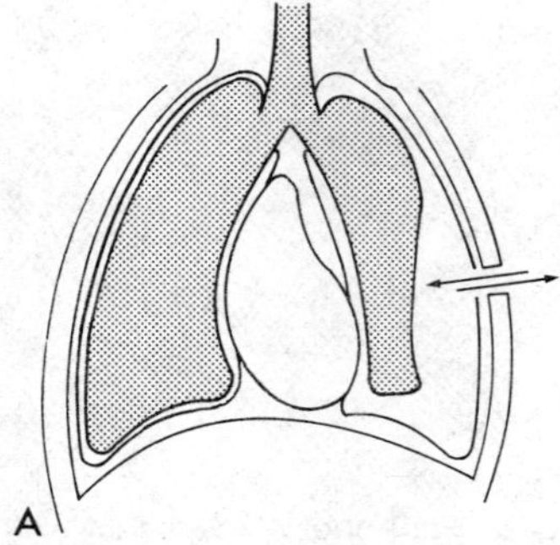

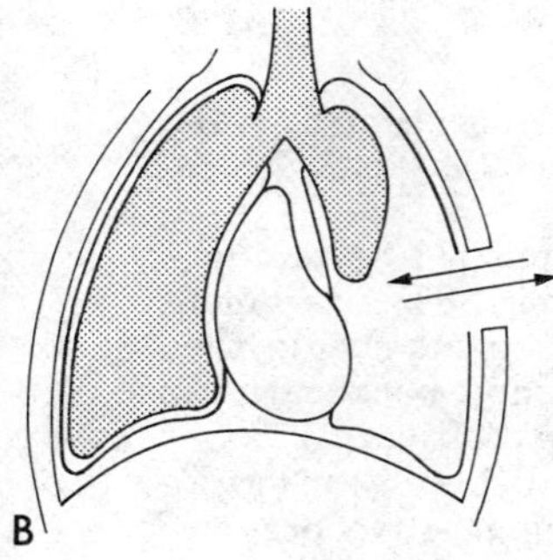

Figure 3–6   Open pneumothorax.

expand, reducing the amount of air taken in on each respiratory movement. Further accumulation of air increasingly restricts lung expansion (Fig. 3–6B).

Spontaneous pneumothorax may occur without the presence of external trauma. It can occur when any other pathological condition allows an alveolus or tracheal bronchus to open into the pleural space.

Traumatic pneumothorax may by produced directly by a penetrating injury or indirectly by blunt trauma. Blunt trauma is the most common cause of pneumothorax. Associated with blunt trauma, but far less common, is a fractured rib penetrating the pleura and lacerating the pulmonary parenchyma beneath.

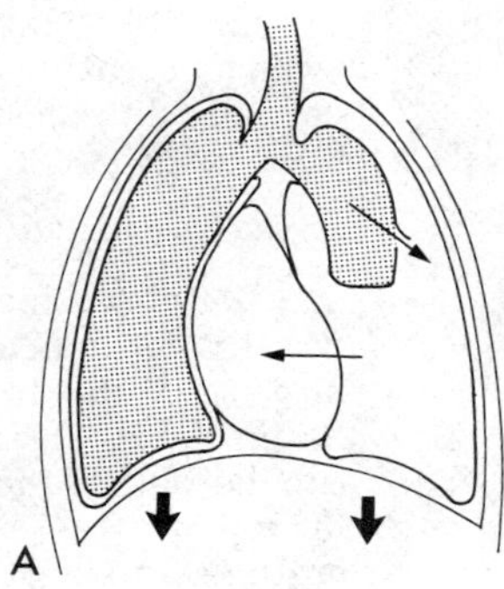

Figure 3–7 Closed pneumothorax.

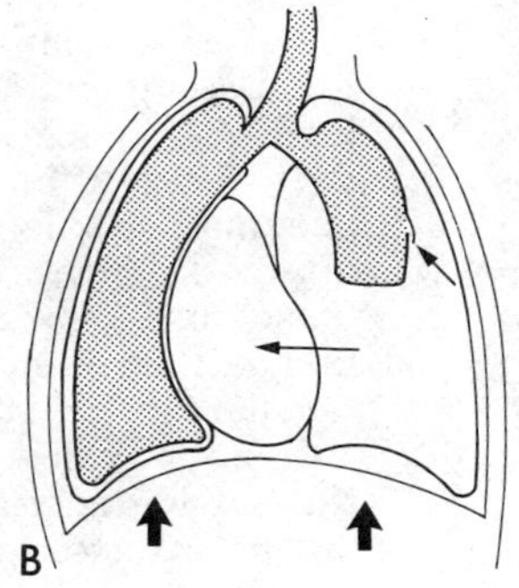

Tension pneumothorax occurs when air enters the pleural space but cannot return either into the alveolus from which it came or to the external environment (Fig. 3–7). An increasing volume of air accumulates. As the volume increases there is an increase of pressure on the lung. When the entire pleural space on one side fills with air, there is a shift of the mediastinum toward the uninvolved side. This produces (1) reduction of lung volume on the uninvolved side, further reducing the movement of air and gaseous exchange and increasing the level of hypoxia; and (2) kinking of the vena cava, restricting blood return to the right atrium and increasing central venous pressure. Because cardiac output and oxygen absorption both fall, tension pneumothorax is rapidly fatal if undiagnosed.

The signs of pneumothorax are (1) absent breath sounds, (2) deviation of the trachea away from the side without breath sounds, (3) cyanosis, (4) distended neck veins, and (5) possible subcutaneous emphysema.

Management of Pneumothorax

Definitive management of *simple pneumothorax* is usually not indicated in the field because accurate diagnosis is difficult without x-ray examination. In the hospital, the presence and location of the pneumothorax can be determined by physical examination and confirmed by x-ray examination. There are two methods of on-the-scene treatment of pneumothorax: (1) insertion of a pneumothorax device with an attached one-way flutter valve, or (2) connecting a patient to waterseal suction.

Decompression of *tension pneumothorax* is accomplished by inserting a needle, a special pneumothorax device with a flutter valve, or a chest tube. In general, pneumothorax is relieved by a tube through the second intercostal space at the midclavicular line, whereas hemothorax (see following) is drained laterally at the mid-axillary line at about the sixth or seventh intercostal space.

One-way flow of air from within the pleural space to the outside is necessary. A large-bore straight needle may be inserted in the second interspace. While a flutter

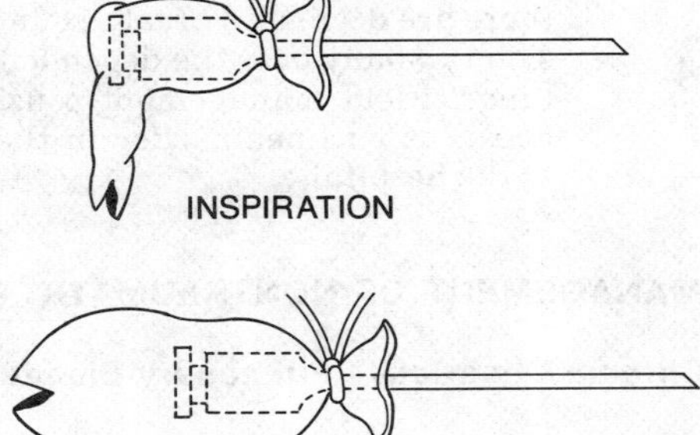

Figure 3–8 A one-way flutter valve attached to a large-bore needle, used for decompression of a tension pneumothorax.

valve is being arranged, a finger covers the end of the needle on inspiration, when thoracic pressure for inspiration is negative. On expiration, when pressure is positive, the finger is removed. A one-way flutter valve can be made by using a finger cot or the finger of a rubber glove with a small hole cut in the end (Fig. 3–8). The hole should be small and the finger cot long to take advantage of external pressure to close the valve on inspiration. One-way flutter valves are available commercially. In the emergency department, one-way flow of air can be assured by an underwater seal and bottle arrangement.

Hemothorax

Hemothorax is most commonly produced when a fractured rib lacerates its associated intercostal artery in blunt trauma, although penetration of the rib into lung tissue or the major pulmonary vasculature can also cause intrathoracic bleeding. In penetrating trauma, either lung tissue or an injured vessel produces the accumulation of blood.

The diagnosis of hemothorax is suspected when there are decreased breath sounds and decreased percussion tympany over the dependent segment of one or both lungs. Field management consists of protection of the chest, as outlined earlier in the chapter, and transport to the hospital.

MANAGEMENT OF NONTRAUMATIC CONDITIONS

Chronic Obstructive Pulmonary Disease

Chronic obstructive pulmonary disease is recognized by a chest expanded (or near expanded) to its maximum in a resting condition. Breathing is by the accessory respiratory muscles and the diaphragm. A person in such distress will frequently place his forearms on his knees to raise the shoulders and allow the accessory muscles more effective thoracic expansion. The patient will frequently be exhaling slowly through pursed lips. As the patient frequently discovers accidentally, this maintains a higher intrapulmonary pressure, allowing complete evacuation of the alveoli despite the collapse of distal bronchi. Inspiratory and expiratory wheezes may or may not be present, as is true of inspiratory rales.

In the pre-hospital phase, chronic obstructive pulmonary disease is treated by low-flow oxygen to partially supplement the patient's oxygen needs. Because the patient has become accustomed to a low level of arterial oxygen, oxygen flows in the range of 6 to 8 liters per minute may trigger a cessation of respiration. If this occurs, immediate intubation and positive pressure ventilation of the patient should be accomplished.

Asthma

Asthma can be diagnosed by frequent supraclavicular, suprasternal, intercostal, and subcostal retraction on inspiration and severe anxiety on the part of the patient, secondary to an inability to move air appropriately. Auscultation reveals bilateral muscial wheezes and shallow respiration. A history of asthma is most helpful in diagnosis.

Asthma attacks may be mild, involving only a few bronchi and bronchioles; or they may be quite severe, with extensive involvement of the entire lung but without associated respiratory distress. These patients, although not requiring aggressive treatment initially, can deteriorate if not adequately managed.

Under physician control, aminophylline (250 to 500 mg IV) is given over a period of 5 to 20 minutes. Steroid dosage (e.g., dexamethasone) begins at 0.2 mg/kg and can reach as high as 2.0 mg/kg. Bronchodilators, such as isoproterenol (Isuprel), may be given by inhalation. Positive pressure ventilation with a high oxygen flow rate is considered primary treatment by some and adjunctive therapy by others.

Pulmonary Edema

Pulmonary edema is seen in patients with decompensated chronic *cardiac* disease, in certain *drug abuses*, and at high altitudes. In mild cases a few moist rales will be heard. As pulmonary edema progresses in severity, there will be severe shortness of breath, frothy sputum and bronchial secretions, and venous congestion in the face and neck.

Treatment is divided into two phases. The initial phase is directed at increasing the level of oxygen in the alveoli and decreasing the patient's oxygen demands. Increased air in the alveoli is accomplished by having the patient breathe high-flow oxygen from nasal prongs or a non-rebreathing bag. Decreasing the patient's anxiety is accomplished by getting the patient, as quickly as possible, into a position of comfort (usually semi-sitting), reassuring him, and trying to get him to slow his respiratory movement and decrease his anxiety.

The second phase of treatment is reducing the amount of edema in the lungs. The first step in this management stage is to apply rotating tourniquets. These venous tourniquets are applied to three of the four extremities with one rotation every five minutes. This method uses venous tourniquet elevation on one extremity for 15 minutes before it is rested for five. Medication can also be used in the management of pulmonary edema but should be utilized only by the EMT-Paramedic or those trained in the pharmacological aspects of patient care.

Pneumonia

Pneumonia is recognized by an elevated temperature; unilateral or bilateral decreased breath sounds; dullness on percussion; and, in severe cases, coughing with bloody sputum, cyanosis, and pulmonary distress. The field treatment of pneumonia consists of oxygen at 6 to 8 liters per minute and intravenous lactated Ringer's solution, 250 ml/hr. Results of sputum cultures will determine appropriate antibiotic therapy.

Atelectasis

Atelectasis is most frequently found in the postoperative surgical patient and is recognized by an elevated temperature and diminished breath sounds. Outside the hospital atelectasis may occur in patients with fractured ribs and other forms of chest trauma. The cause is usually a mucous plug in the bronchi due to decreased respiratory excursions. Encouraging deep, hard coughing is frequently effective in removing a mucous plug.

SPECIAL PROBLEMS

Fractured Larynx

Direct trauma to the larynx can produce fractures that significantly compromise respiration. The diagnosis of these unusual results of trauma is easy to miss. The symptoms of a fractured larynx are hoarseness, palpable loss of continuity of the laryngeal box, and subcutaneous emphysema. A fractured larynx is managed conservatively if possible. If the airway is compromised, endo-tracheal intubation is the treatment of choice. Cri-cothyroidotomy or tracheostomy may be utilized if endotracheal intubation is not possible.

Acute Bronchial Obstruction

Acute bronchial obstruction is recognized by absent or decreased breath sounds on one side of the chest. Deviation of the trachea toward that side distinguishes bronchial obstruction from tension pneumothorax, in which there is deviation away from the side of absent breath sounds. An obstruction in the bronchus allows the escape of air but does not allow alveolar filling. The other lung overexpands, with shifting of the mediastinum toward the obstruction. Bronchial obstruction is not usually as severe as tension pneumothorax.

Pre-hospital management is limited to reassurance and possible sedation of the patient, with oxygen admin-istration.

Acute Bronchial Spasm

This condition, although similar to asthma, is usual-ly secondary to an acute allergic reaction, which may rapidly progress to anaphylactic shock. Distinguishing features are high-pitched wheezes; difficult respiration; intercostal, substernal, and subcostal retraction; and cyanosis. Allergic conditions that produce severe bron-chospasm and laryngospasm require 0.1 to 0.5 ml of 1:1000 epinephrine subcutaneously. Positive pressure ventilation is effective.

Face and Neck Injuries

Management of respiratory problems arising from extensive injuries to the face and neck is discussed in Chapter 7.

shock

A patient is in shock when, for any reason, there is inadequate perfusion of oxygen and nutrient materials to the cells of the body. Failure to improve perfusion leads to the progressive death of cells, impaired organ function, and, ultimately, death of the patient.

TYPES OF SHOCK

Hypovolemic shock is caused by a decrease in effective blood volume. A blood volume deficit of 15 to 25 per cent will usually cause a fall in systolic blood pressure; a blood volume deficit of more than 45 per cent is usually fatal. Shock following trauma is usually of the hypovolemic type, caused either by bleeding (external or internal) or by fluid loss into contused tissue or distended bowel. Damage to the heart or lungs can also contribute significantly to the problem. Shock from excessive fluid loss also occurs in extensively burned patients.

Cardiogenic shock is caused by impaired function of the heart as a pump as in acute myocardial infarction, cardiac tamponade, or pulmonary embolism or following open heart surgery. Arrhythmias can also greatly reduce cardiac output and blood pressure.

Septic shock results from infection. The hyperdynamic type, in which there is normal or increased cardiac output, occurs when the blood volume is adequate but the infection interferes with cell metabolism so that tissue cells cannot adequately utilize the glucose and oxygen carried to them by the blood. In the hypodynamic type the patients have become hypovolemic, usually owing to leakage of fluid from capillaries into the interstitial spaces. Occasionally blood volume is normal, but vascular capacity is increased, causing a relative hypovolemia.

Neurogenic shock is produced by interference with the sympathetic nervous system, causing dilation of arterioles and increased vascular capacity. The systolic blood pressure will usually fall below 80 to 90 mm Hg in spite of normal or increased cardiac output. Ordinary fainting is an example of transient neurogenic shock. Damage to the cervical spinal cord is the most common cause of traumatic neurogenic shock.

Trauma to the brain itself almost never causes shock. As a matter of fact, it almost invariably leads to a rise in blood pressure. Severe head trauma usually increases intracranial pressure and reduces cerebral perfusion. This reflexly stimulates the vasomotor center to increase peripheral vasoconstriction and blood pressure. In the very late stages of brain death, hypotension due to dysfunction of the vasomotor center in the medulla may occur, but only after spontaneous respirations have also ceased.

Anaphylactic shock is caused by a massive release of histamine and other vasoactive agents from cells that have been previously sensitized to specific substances such as penicillin, bee stings, or shellfish. Sudden cardiovascular collapse with or without respiratory dysfunction or airway obstruction due to bronchoconstriction, angioneurotic edema, or urticaria of the airway is not uncommon.

Other important types of shock include those due to drug overdose and hypoglycemia. Barbiturate overdose is particularly apt to cause hypotension and ventilatory depression. The hypotension is caused by a relative hypovolemia due to an increase in capacity and, possibly, some myocardial suppression in the most severe cases. Although the blood pressure is low, skin perfusion appears to be adequate because the blood vessels in the skin are dilated.

Insulin or *hypoglycemic shock* should always be considered in individuals who are in shock but do not clearly fall into the other categories, particularly if there is any suspicion that the patient is a diabetic. The patient may initially be very confused and tends to have cold clammy skin and tachycardia. Administration of glucose produces profound rapid improvement.

DIAGNOSIS OF SHOCK

The respiratory rate is usually quite rapid in patients in shock. Because of the reduced cardiac output and vasoconstriction, the skin is usually cool and pale but the mucous membranes and nail beds may be cyanotic. Excessive sympathetic stimulation causes secretion of sweat, resulting in a clammy skin. The pulse is usually weak and rapid, often barely detectable. The systolic blood pressure is usually low and in severe shock is often not detectable at all. The blood pressure tends to improve slightly if an upright patient lies down and worsens if a prone patient tries to sit up. The arterial pulse pressure (systolic-diastolic) reflects changes in stroke volume and usually falls long before the systolic pressure falls. Urine output is usually decreased or absent. The sensorium tends to be clouded very early, and these patients are usually confused, apprehensive, and restless. Thirst is common, particularly if the patient is questioned.

In hyperdynamic septic shock, neurogenic shock, and barbiturate shock and in occasional patients with acute myocardial infarction shock, the skin may be warm and dry. In neurogenic shock and occasionally in acute myocardial infarction shock, the pulse rate may be relatively slow.

IMMEDIATE TREATMENT

1. Ensure an adequate airway and begin oxygen at 3 to 5 liter/min. Make sure that the minute ventilation is normal or increased.

2. Obtain vital signs and start a flow sheet that includes these and timing of all fluids, drugs, and other treatment.

3. If the patient is hypovolemic, elevate the legs to a 45-degree angle to obtain a rapid return of venous blood from the legs to the heart. When fluids cannot be given immediately and the patient is severely hypotensive, raising both legs to a 90-degree angle further increases venous return. The head and chest should be kept level, otherwise the viscera will press on the diaphragm and impair ventilation. Even better return of venous blood is achieved by the use of air splints or anti-shock garments.

4. Start a rapid infusion of lactated Ringer's solution or normal saline using one or two 18-gauge or larger IV catheters or needles. If an adult is obviously hypovolemic, 1000 to 2000 ml of fluid can usually be given safely over a period of 20 to 40 minutes. In a child, an intravenous push of 10 ml per pound is usually safe.

5. If available, cardioscope leads should be applied to the patient to obtain a continuous EKG reading.

6. Qualified EMT-Paramedics should insert an indwelling urinary catheter if travel time to the emergency department will exceed two hours.

7. In specific circumstances and under a physician's directions, qualified EMT-Paramedics may administer certain drugs such as glucose for suspected hypoglycemia, lidocaine for frequent premature ventricular contraction or ventricular tachycardia, or epinephrine for possible anaphylactic shock.

8. An anti-shock (MAST) garment may be particularly helpful in hypovolemic patients who must be transported a long distance.

ANTI-SHOCK TROUSERS

Anti-shock trousers (MAST) consist of inflatable units that exert pressure on the lower extremities and abdomen, forcing blood into the heart, brain, and lung circulation for the initial management of hypovolemic shock. They are also useful in the management of hemorrhage and fractures.

In hypovolemic shock not enough fluid is presented to the heart to perfuse through body tissue, bringing oxygen and nutrients to the cells. The anti-shock trousers apply pressure to the lower extremities, thus decreasing container size (blood vessel volume) and increasing peripheral resistance. The available blood is therefore shunted upward to support the more oxygen-sensitive organs — the heart, brain, and lungs. Up to 2000 ml of blood can be thus relocated in this autotransfusion.

The absolute indication for the application of anti-shock trousers in hypovolemic shock is a systolic blood pressure below 80 mm Hg. A relative indication is a blood pressure below 100 mg Hg. The difference depends on the size, sex, and age of the patient. Elderly patients, particularly small, elderly females, can run a normal systolic pressure of between 80 and 100 mm Hg. It would be inappropriate to apply anti-shock trousers to these patients, particularly if other signs and symptoms of shock are not present.

Application of Trousers

It is most appropriate to move the patient from his position in his bed or inside the automobile onto the opened pneumatic counter compression device on the ambulance gurney. Such prior planning by the EMT or the physician in the emergency department can speed the application of MAST trousers as well as prevent unnecessary movement of the patient. If for some reason the trousers have not been applied, they can rapidly be slipped beneath the patient by two individuals. One individual stands on each side of the patient and with the cephalad (head) hand grasps the trousers and with the caudad (foot) hand elevates the feet. The trousers are then slipped to the level of the buttocks. With the cephalad hand remaining on the trousers, the caudad hand grasps the patient's belt or buttocks, elevates the hip region and slides the trousers to the level of the lower rib cage. The garment is secured by pressing together the Velcro fasteners, first around the legs and then around the abdomen. The genitalia are left exposed so that Foley catheterization may be performed. Stopcocks are placed in the open position and the foot pump is used to inflate the garment until the patient's pressure returns to within normal limits. It must be emphasized that the pressure within the garment is unimportant. The patient is in shock, not the trousers. Therefore, attention should be directed to the patient and elevating his pressure and not to the unimportant pressure within the garment itself.

One of the disadvantages of inflating the abdominal section is decreased respiratory excursion and hypoventilation, caused by the increased abdominal pressure. If assisted ventilation is used, this disadvantage is neutralized.

Deflation of the Trousers

Once the garment has been placed on a patient who is in shock, it should not be deflated and removed until the proper equipment, personnel, and setting are available for whole-blood replacement and operative repair of the traumatized area.

Just as the constriction about the legs and abdomen decreases the size of the container and allows more blood to flow in the upper part of the body, so deflation of the garment increases the size of the container and deprives the upper part of the body, particularly the heart, brain, and lung circulation, of this extra fluid load. Failure to replace the fluid when the container has been expanded will return the patient to his previous shocklike state unless the body's defense mechanisms produce enough epinephrine and norepinephrine to constrict these vessels internally.

If possible, deflation of the garment should proceed in the hospital under the direction of a physician. All personnel included in caring for a patient on whom an anti-shock garment has been used must be thoroughly familiar with all aspects of its use. The abdomen should be gradually deflated a small increment at a time with constant attention to the blood pressure. If the blood pressure drops as much as 5 mm Hg systolic, deflation should stop and fluid should be replaced in the expanding container until the blood pressure returns to within normal limits. After it has returned to within normal limits deflation can be continued. As much as 2000 ml of fluid may have to be administered as the garment is being deflated.

If the possibility of intraabdominal blood loss exists, such as would be present with a ruptured spleen or liver, or a dissecting aortic aneurysm, deflation should not be attempted until the patient is in the operating room and prepared for a laparotomy. At this time deflation can be accomplished and the abdomen rapidly opened to prevent further unnecessary blood loss.

Contraindications

The contraindications to the use of anti-shock garments are situations in which a rapid autotransfusion of blood volume from the lower half of the body to the central circulation might aggravate the patient's condition. In closed head injuries, an increase in central blood volume tends to increase intracranial pressure and could have disastrous results. Patients who have pulmonary edema or congestive heart failure will also be made worse by the anti-shock garment. In addition, trauma involving only the head, neck, chest, or upper extremities with internal hemorrhage or other bleeding that cannot be controlled by applying direct pressure to the bleeding point may be aggravated by an anti-shock garment. In fact, an autotransfusion from the lower extremities might result in increased hemorrhage rather than effective restoration of blood volume.

MONITORING

Monitoring of blood pressure, heart rate, and rhythm, and respiratory rate and depth must be continuous. Changes in *pulse pressure* reflect changes in the stroke volume of the heart and thus are better indicators of blood flow than systolic pressure. If a patient has cold and clammy *skin,* it can generally be assumed that his cardiac output is low and his peripheral vascular resistance is high. A clouded *sensorium* is evidence of poor tissue perfusion. If the urine output is low and falling it can be assumed that renal perfusion is reduced or inadequate for proper kidney function.

Urine output is measured at least hourly by an EMT if transport time to the emergency department will exceed two hours. In the hospital an intraarterial catheter may be used to measure blood pressure, and central venous pressure and serial blood gas determinations should be obtained as well.

The flow sheet with an accurate indication of all vital signs and treatment is the basis of all monitoring.

cardiovascular emergencies

Cardiovascular emergencies often involve heart attack or cardiac arrest. The following sections on basic life support and advanced life support have been excerpted and condensed with permission from the American Heart Association from their manuals for instructors of basic and advanced cardiac life support.

Emergency cardiac care includes the following elements: (1) recognizing the early warning signs of heart attack, preventing complications, reassuring the victim, and moving him to a life-support unit without delay; (2) providing immediate basic life support at the scene when needed; (3) providing advanced life support as quickly as possible; and (4) transferring the stabilized victim for continued cardiac care.

BASIC CARDIAC LIFE SUPPORT (BCLS)

Basic cardiac life support is that phase of emergency cardiac care that either externally supports the circulation and respiration of the cardiac arrest victim through cardiopulmonary resuscitation, or prevents circulatory or respiratory arrest or insufficiency through prompt intervention. Any trained person can apply basic cardiac life support.

Each year heart attacks account for over 350,000 deaths that occur before the victim reaches the hospital. Many of these deaths could have been prevented if someone had immediately come to the victim's aid, preferably within the first two minutes after the onset signal. The usual cause of death in heart attacks is electrical instability of the heart, which begins at the onset of myocardial injury. Sudden death or cardiac arrest (the abrupt, unexpected cessation of breathing and circulation) may occur as the initial or only manifestation of coronary artery disease, especially during a heart attack.

Cardiac arrest, which is recognized by an absence of pulse, can result from the following:

1. Ventricular fibrillation, when there is a chaotic, uncoordinated twitching of the individual fibers of the myocardium but no cardiac contraction;

2. Ventricular standstill (asystole), when there is neither electrical activity nor cardiac contraction; or

3. Cardiovascular collapse (electromechanical dissociation), when there is evidence of electrical activity but ineffective cardiac muscle contraction.

These electrical mechanisms, all of which result in an absence of pulse, can only be differentiated from one another by an electrocardiogram. The initial treatment for all of these is cardiopulmonary resuscitation.

Within seconds after a cardiac arrest occurs, the victim loses consciousness and stops breathing. During this early phase the victim may have a convulsion. Within 30 seconds the pupils sometimes become widely dilated. The sooner circulation to the brain is restored, the greater the chance for full recovery of brain function. Significant brain damage usually occurs after four to six minutes of cardiac arrest. Children, especially infants, and victims of drowning and cold exposure may recover normal brain function after longer periods of cardiac arrest. The infant's brain is more resistant to injury from a lack of oxygen; victims of drowning and cold exposure may be protected by their lower body temperature. Any individual who has sustained cardiac arrest may be kept alive with basic cardiac life support.

Signs of cardiac arrest are unconsciousness, absence

of respiratory movements, and no pulsations in the carotid or femoral arteries. Cardiopulmonary resuscitation is begun by first establishing the patient's unresponsiveness. The rescuer should gently shake the shoulder of the victim and ask, "Are you okay?" If the victim does not respond to attempts to arouse him, call out for help. Position the patient on his back. To protect the neck from possible cervical injuries, carefully turn the entire body as one unit. The rescuer should kneel at the side of the victim.

Since the tongue is the most common cause of airway obstruction in the unconscious victim, the airway frequently may be opened simply by utilizing the head tilt method. The rescuer places one hand beneath the victim's neck and the other hand on the forehead. The neck is then lifted with one hand while tilting the head by backward pressure on the forehead with the other hand (see Fig. 3–1). If there is a possibility of cervical neck injury, such as after a diving or automobile accident, the head tilt method is not utilized. The jaw thrust method is much safer. In the jaw thrust method, the rescuer grasps the angles of the victim's lower jaw, one hand on each side of the head over the ears, and, lifting with both hands, displaces the mandible forward while tilting the head backward. The airway can usually be opened without extending the neck.

While maintaining the open airway position, the rescuer places his ear over the victim's mouth and nose, looking toward the victim's chest and stomach and watching for movement, listening for air escaping during exhalation, and feeling for the flow of air on the cheek. If the victim is not breathing, rescue breathing must be applied.

The best way to provide rescue breathing is by using the mouth-to-mouth technique. Take the hand that is on the victim's forehead and turn it so that you can pinch the victim's nose shut while keeping the heel of the hand on the forehead to maintain the tilt of the head. The other hand should remain under the victim's neck (or chin), lifting up. Initially give four quick full breaths without allowing time for full lung deflation between breaths. Adequate volumes required in an adult to see the chest rise are usually in the range of 800 to 1200 ml of air. This is usually equivalent to a double size breath of the rescuer.

The presence or absence of a pulse is then determined by palpating for the carotid pulse. To find the carotid artery, take the hand that is under the victim's neck and locate the voice box. Slide the tips of the index fingers into the groove beside the voice box. If the pulse is present, the rescuer continues to perform rescue breathing, ventilating the lungs once every five seconds until help arrives. If the pulse is absent, artificial circulation must be provided in addition to rescue breathing. This is cardiopulmonary resuscitation, or CPR.

With the victim in the horizontal position, the rescuer locates the lower margin of the victim's rib cage on the side next to the rescuer with the middle and index fingers of the lower hand. The fingers are then run up along the rib cage to the notch where the ribs meet the sternum in the center of the lower chest. With one finger on the notch, the other finger is placed next to the first finger on the lower end of the sternum. The heel of the other hand is placed on the lower half of the sternum. The long axis of the heel of the hand should be placed on the long axis of the breast bone. The first hand is then removed from the notch and placed on top of the hand on the sternum so that both hands are parallel and directed straight down from the rescuer (Fig. 5–1A). The fingers must be held away from the chest wall (Fig. 5–1B). The rescuer's shoulders are positioned directly over his hands, and the elbows are locked so that the thrust for external heart compression is straight down. To achieve the most pressure with the least amount of effort, the rescuer leans forward until his shoulders are directly over his outstretched hands and the breast bone of the victim (Fig. 5–1C).

To compress the sternum of a normal size adult, enough force to depress the sternum 1½ to 2 in must be exerted. With each compression the heart must be squeezed sufficiently to pump blood through the body. When the pressure is released the heart is allowed to refill. When performing CPR alone, compressions must be done in this manner at a rate of 80 times per minute.

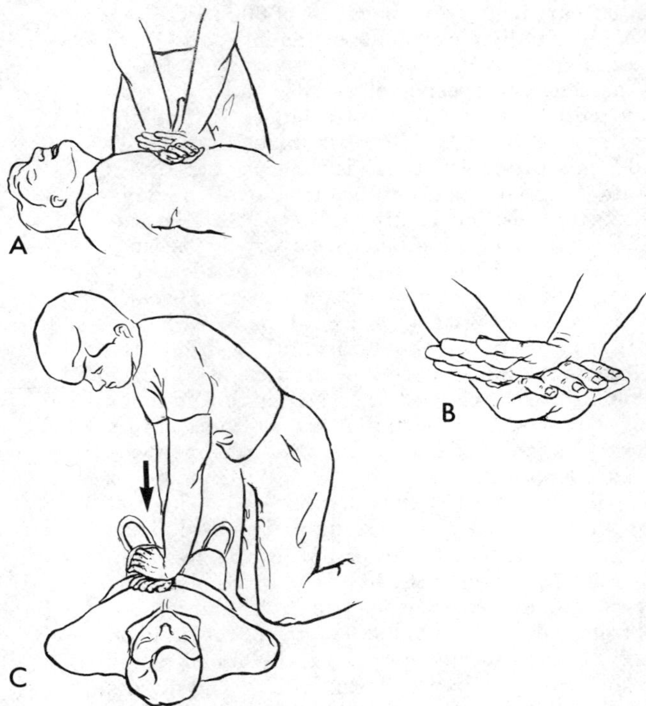

Figure 5–1 External cardiac compression.

The ratio of compression to relaxation when performing external cardiac compression is approximately two-thirds of the time spent in compression and one-third of the time spent in relaxation (2:1). During relaxation the hands should not be lifted off the chest or their position changed in any way because correct hand position may be lost. Bouncing compressions must be avoided, since they are less effective and are more likely to cause injury.

If there is only one rescuer, 15 cardiac compressions must be performed at a rate of 80 times per minute. Following the 15 compressions, two quick full ventilations must be delivered. The rescuer then moves back to the chest, locates the proper hand position, and begins 15 compressions at a rate of 80 per minute again (Table 5–1).

If available, a second rescuer should take over ventilation. The second rescuer is positioned on the opposite side of the victim and interposes a breath during the upstroke of any chest compression. With two rescuers, only 60 compressions per minute need to be given, because the compressions will not need to be interrupted. The first rescuer should utilize a mnemonic of "1-1000, 2-1000, 3-1000, 4-1000, 5-1000," in order for the second rescuer to interpose a ventilation during the upstroke of each fifth chest compression. There should be no pause or hesitation between the fifth compression and the first compression of the next cycle of five. The ventilator should feel for the carotid pulse frequently during chest compression to assess the effectiveness of compression.

Ventilation and compression should be interrupted periodically (every four to five minutes) to check for the return of spontaneous breathing and pulse. Cardiopulmonary resuscitation should never be interrupted for more than five seconds except in special situations, at which time it may be interrupted for no more than 15 seconds.

When performing CPR with two rescuers, they may change positions using the following procedure: the chest compressor, instead of saying "1-1000, 2-1000, 3-1000, 4-1000, 5-1000," says "Change on 3 next time." This signals the rescue breather that the chest compressor is tired and wishes to change positions. After delivering the next ventilation, the rescue breather moves down the

Table 5–1 COMPRESSION AND BREATH RATES IN CPR

No. of Rescuers	Ratio of Compressions to Breaths	Rates of Compression (times/min)
1	15:2	80
2	5:1	60

side of the victim opposite the chest compressor. With the middle and index fingers of one hand the rescue breather locates the lower margin of the victim's rib cage on the side opposite the chest compressor. When the chest compressor has completed the third compression, the rescue breather slides his hands from below onto the sternum into the proper position, sweeping the compressor's hands off the chest. He should pick up compressions 4 and 5. The chest compressor, who must not leave the chest until his hands are pushed off, moves directly to rescue breathing, interposing a breath during the up-stroke of the fifth chest compression.

p. 26
p. 57

Do not attempt external cardiac compression in patients with severe crushing injuries of the chest, suspected **tension pneumothorax**, severe emphysema, or suspected **cardiac tamponade**. Thoracotomy, manual cardiac compression, and drainage may be necessary in the emergency department.

Infants and Small Children

When treating infants and small children, it is important to remember the following differences.

When clearing the airway of an infant, be careful that you do not exaggerate the backward position of the head tilt. An infant's neck is so pliable that forceful backward tilting may block breathing passages instead of opening them.

During artificial respiration, do not try to pinch the nose. Cover both the mouth and nose of an infant or small child who is not breathing. Use small breaths with less volume to inflate the lungs. Give one small breath every three seconds.

The absence of a pulse may be easily determined in an infant or child by feeling over the left nipple.

When performing chest compression on infants and small children, use only one hand. The other hand may be slipped under the child to provide a firm support for his back. For infants, use only the tips of the index and middle fingers to compress the chest at mid-sternum. Depress the sternum between 1/2 and 3/4 in at a fast rate of 80 to 100 times per minute. For small children, use only the heel of one hand to compress the chest. Depress the sternum between 3/4 and 1½ in depending on the size of the child. The rate should be 80 to 100 times per minute.

Breaths should be administered during relaxation after every fifth chest compression for both infants and small children.

ADVANCED LIFE SUPPORT

Advanced life support is one component of emergency cardiac care and consists of more than definitive therapy for the patient in cardiac arrest. Advanced life support serves a preventive role for the patient who has sustained a myocardial infarction and has a high risk of cardiac arrest. The majority of resuscitable cardiac arrest patients are those individuals whose arrests follow an acute myocardial infarction. The arrest probably occurs within the first two hours following the acute episode, and it is now understood that the etiology of the arrest is most frequently and initially of the mildest rhythm disorder, progressing to a fatal arrhythmia.

Any patient sustaining a possible myocardial infarction or under cardiopulmonary emergency care should have his cardiac rhythm and rate monitored on an oscilloscope. An intravenous infusion should be established using D_5W. This will allow medication such as atropine for bradycardia or lidocaine for premature ventricular contraction to be administered, since these arrhythmias may signal impending cardiac arrest. By visually monitoring the cardiac rhythm and rate, the development of ventricular tachycardia, ventricular fibrillation, or asystole can be rapidly recognized and appropriate therapy instituted immediately. The administration of prophylactic lidocaine to prevent the development of arrhythmias that have a fatal outcome is being utilized. Early cardiac care frequently prevents the need for all CPR. Appropriate patient monitoring also allows for early recognition and treatment of pulmonary edema and cardiogenic shock. In the out-of-hospital situation, transportation with continued monitoring may take place when the patient has been stabilized.

When a patient with myocardial infarction develops cardiac arrest, the following elements must be instituted:

1. Basic life support;
2. Use of adjunctive equipment for ventilation and circulation;
3. Cardiac monitoring for arrhythmia recognition and control;
4. Defibrillation;
5. Establishment and maintenance of an intravenous infusion line;
6. Utilization of definitive therapy, including drug administration, for correction of acidosis and for assistance in establishing and maintaining an effective cardiac rhythm and circulation;
7. Stabilization of the patient's condition; and
8. Transportation with continuous monitoring.

Basic life support must be instituted immediately, or the administration of advanced life support is of no value.

Advanced life support can be approached through two main routes: ventilation and perfusion. Ventilation consists of three basic elements: intubation, oxygenation, and ventilation.

Intubation may be achieved either intratracheally by the oral or nasal route or with an esophageal obturator airway. It is necessary to secure and maintain the airway and prevent aspiration. Supplemental oxygenation utilizing 100 per cent oxygen is essential because of the decreased arterial oxygenation that occurs during cardiac arrest from reduced cardiac output and functional residual capacity. Intrapulmonary shunting ventilation is achieved using a self-inflating bag with an oxygen reservoir or other adjunctive ventilatory equipment that will deliver supplemental oxygen.

Restoration of normal circulation is the most essential part of advanced life support. Application of the electrode-defibrillator paddles provides immediate information on the cardiac rhythm (Fig. 5–2). In cardiac arrest the most frequently observed mode is ventricular fibrillation and, occasionally, asystole.

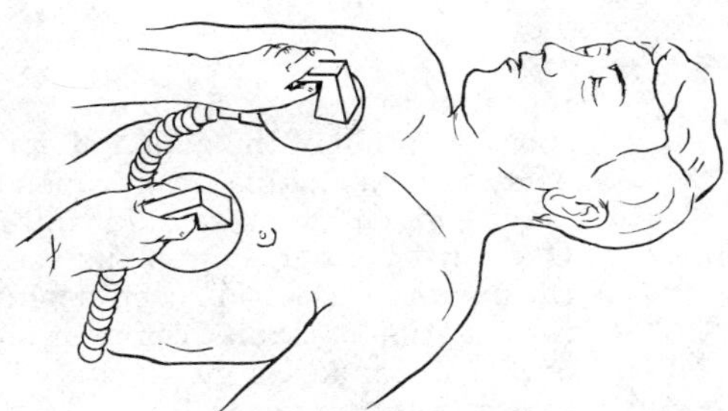

Figure 5–2 Placement of defibrillator paddles.

If ventricular fibrillation is observed, immediate countershock using 3.5 to 6 watt seconds per kilogram is instituted. The paddles should be maintained in place and the cardiac rhythm observed for ventricular fibrillation, normal sinus rhythm, or asystole. The initial application of the paddles, recognition of rhythm, charge and discharge of the defibrillator, and re-recognition of the post-defibrillation rhythm can be achieved in 15 to 20 seconds. Under these circumstances, the need to start an infusion and give drugs first is not indicated, since countershock can be rapidly delivered before excessive hypoxemia or acidosis develops.

If the post-defibrillation rhythm is ventricular fibrillation, asystole, or electromechanical dissociation, continue CPR. Implement intubation, oxygenation, and ventilation and establish an IV infusion with D_5W, using a peripheral vein if possible. If a peripheral vein is not utilized, the femoral or jugular vein may be suitable for cannulation in the hospital. Insertion of the catheter into the subclavian vein during uninterrupted extracardiac compression is extremely difficult.

After securing an intravenous line and infusing fluids, drug therapy should be started. Sodium bicarbonate (1mEq/kg) is given initially to counteract acidosis. Thereafter, half the initial dose can be given at 10-minute intervals, but blood graphs and pH determinations should guide treatment whenever feasible. Epinephrine should also be given in the dose of 0.5 to 1 mg initially by the intravenous route for its alpha- and beta-receptor stimulating actions. It is necessary to repeat this dose at 5-minute intervals because of the short duration of the action of epinephrine. If there is a delay in establishing an intravenous route, epinephrine may be given by intracardiac injection in the same dose. One must be cognizant of the possible hazards of intracardiac administration of epinephrine, which include the interruption of cardiac compression and ventilation, cardiac tamponade, coronary artery laceration, pneumothorax, and intramyocardial injection, which may produce intractable ventricular fibrillation. Epinephrine may also be instilled directly into the tracheobronchial tree and endotracheal tube.

External cardiac compression should be continued to circulate these drugs, and the status of the cardiac rhythm should be reassessed. If ventricular fibrillation is present, the patient should again be defibrillated. If asystole or electromechanical dissociation is present, further drug therapy is indicated. If normal sinus rhythm is seen, check the pulse to see if it is palpable. If normal sinus rhythm returns but with bradycardia and hypotension, atropine administration (0.5 mg IV every five minutes up to a total of 2.0 mg) is indicated.

If ventricular fibrillation is still present or rapid or returns after a very short episode of normal sinus rhythm, sodium bicarbonate and lidocaine are indicated. If fibrillation is fine, epinephrine is also required.

If asystole or electromechanical dissociation persists, continue drug therapy and reassess oxygenation. Drug therapy for asystole and electromechanical dissociation includes calcium chloride and isoproterenol.

In the post-resuscitation stage, a useful drug such as dopamine, metaraminol, and, occasionally, levarterenol may be indicated to support blood pressure. Assessment of oxygenation and acid-base balance may prevent recurrence of cardiac arrest. The need for mechanical ventilation should also be assessed.

ACUTE MYOCARDIAL INFARCTION

Acute myocardial infarction is a serious problem frequently encountered in medicine today. Statistics indicate that some 360,000 persons sustain cardiac arrests from myocardial infarction before they arrive at a hospital. Since the severe complications of cardiac arrest usually occur within the first two hours, it is imperative that the signs and symptoms of an acute myocardial infarction be recognized as quickly as possible.

The patient suffering from an acute myocardial infarction usually complains of severe crushing chest pain substernally. Occasionally the pain may originate in the epigastrium and radiate up into the chest area or upper extremities. If the pain originates midsternally, it frequently radiates down the inner aspect of the left arm. Other symptoms are restlessness, dyspnea, sweating, weakness, nausea, and vomiting. The skin may be cool and clammy and the physical signs of weak rapid pulse, moist basilar rales of the lungs, and an audible diastolic gallop may be present. The signs and symptoms are usually caused by an inadequate coronary artery blood supply due to severe atherosclerosis or thrombosis.

Treatment of a patient suspected of sustaining an acute myocardial infarction involves putting the individual at complete rest. Oxygen is administered at a rate of 4 to 6 liters per minute, preferably by mask or nasal cannula. If signs of congestive heart failure are present, the patient will best tolerate the oxygen by nasal cannula. An accurate history must be taken from the patient, evaluating the chief complaint of chest pain according to location, quality, quantity, duration, associated symptoms, precipitating factors, and alleviating symptoms. Obtain vital signs and note any alteration in blood pressure, pulse rate, and respiratory rate. It is important to note that the initial blood pressure may be elevated due to the patient's response to the pain. The relief of pain may also bring a subsequent drop in blood pressure.

The pain of myocardial infarction usually lasts 20 to 30 minutes and is not relieved by rest or the administration of nitroglycerine. It is imperative that the pain be relieved early in the treatment. This is usually accomplished by the administration of morphine or Demerol. Once analgesics are administered it is important to recheck the blood pressure and other vital signs at frequent 5- to 10-minute intervals because of the subsequent drop in blood pressure as a response to the analgesic. The electrocardiogram should be monitored, and any abnormalities observed should be treated.

As soon as possible a full 12-lead electrocardiogram should be taken to identify the area of infarction and to have a baseline EKG with which to compare subsequent 12-lead EKGs. A routine chest x-ray should be taken as soon as possible to determine such complications as congestive heart failure and pulmonary embolism. Blood should be drawn for CBC, electrolyte determination, and levels of cardiac enzymes creatine phosphokinase (CPK), serum glutamic oxaloacetic transaminase (SGOT), lactic dehydrogenase (LDH), and hydroxybutyrate dehydrogenase (HBD).

If the patient is restless, treatment with sedatives should be initiated early to ensure rest and relieve anxiety. Medications such as phenobarbital (30 mg), chlordiazepoxide hydrochloride (Librium, 10 mg), or diazepam (Valium, 2 to 5 mg) in divided daily dosages may help.

Complications of Acute Myocardial Infarction

Arrhythmias

Arrhythmias following acute myocardial infarction are frequent and varied in type. Frequently encountered arrhythmias include premature ventricular contractions, bradycardia, rapid atrial fibrillation, A-V blocks, ventricular tachycardia, and the lethal arrhythmias of ventricular fibrillation and asystole.

PREMATURE VENTRICULAR CONTRACTIONS. These contractions are common and may be a response to the insult to the myocardium. They may also be a sign of hypoxia. If they remain after the initiation of oxygen therapy, they must be reevaluated as to their clinical significance. If the premature ventricular contractions are multifocal in nature, are occurring with a frequency of greater than six per minute, or are occurring in salvos, they may be precursors of a more serious ventricular arrhythmia such as ventricular tachycardia or ventricular fibrillation. If they are deemed to be clinically significant, it is recommended that a bolus of lidocaine of 50 to 100 mg be given by intravenous push. This should be followed by a lidocaine infusion of 2 to 4 mg/min. The lidocaine drip should be titrated according to the patient's response and the relief of the premature ventricular contractions. Caution should be taken that no more than 300 mg of lidocaine be given in the first hour.

BRADYCARDIA. Because of parasympathetic stimulation resulting from the myocardial infarction, patients may present with bradycardia. If the pulse rate is below 60 per minute and there is associated hypotension, drug therapy with atropine (0.5 to 1.0 mg IV) is indicated. If the clinical symptoms of hypotension and poor cerebral profusion remain without an increase in the pulse rate, it may be necessary to start an isoproterenol drip of 1 mg in 500 ml of D_5W. This should be instituted with a small minidrip IV administration set and initially started at 20 to 30 minidrips per minute. The initial infusion rate will depend on the patient's response. It must be pointed out that isoproterenol increases myocardial oxygen demands and may extend the area of infarction. Since isoproterenol is also a beta-receptor stimulating drug, tachyarrhythmias may result from its administration.

ATRIAL VENTRICULAR (A-V) BLOCKS. These blocks are a frequent complication of myocardial infarction. A first degree block, which is a prolongation of the PR interval beyond 0.2 seconds, should be observed but is usually not treated. A second degree A-V block (Mobitz Type I) shows an increasing prolongation of the PR interval until a QRS complex is dropped. Again, individuals sustaining a Mobitz Type I A-V block should be monitored closely, since this is usually an indication of more serious blocks to come. However, the Mobitz Type I block is usually not treated unless there is frequent dropping of the QRS complex with resulting clinical symptoms of hypotension and decreased cerebral perfusion. If these symptoms are present, the individual may receive 0.5 to 1.0 mg of atropine intravenously to a total of 2.0 mg.

Mobitz Type II block is a more serious arrhythmia because of its frequent dropping of the QRS complex. In a Mobitz Type II block the PR interval remains constant with a periodic dropping of the QRS complex on either a variable or a cyclic pattern. Individuals sustaining a Mobitz Type II block frequently have symptoms of decreasing cardiac output and will require treatment with atropine in the dosages previously mentioned.

Third degree or complete heart block may be evident following an acute myocardial infarction. In this particular rhythm there is no coordination between the atrial and ventricular contractions. Since the inherent rate of the ventricles is around 20 to 40 per minute, the patient frequently presents with signs of poor cardiac output such as hypotension and poor cerebral perfusion. Atropine (0.5 to 1.0 mg) may be given by IV push. If there is no increase in rate in response to atropine, an isoproterenol drip of 1 mg in 500 small ml D_5W may be started in an attempt to increase the ventricular rate. Individuals presenting with third degree or complete heart block need to have a pacemaker inserted to ensure adequate cardiac output.

RAPID ATRIAL FIBRILLATION. Atrial fibrillation may be a frequent finding in the patient suffering from acute myocardial infarction. There is very little that can be done in the field for this arrhythmia besides elective countershock. This procedure must be used with extreme caution in patients on digitalis preparations. The danger of this arrhythmia is that it promotes clot formation in the atria that may then break off emboli to other parts of the body.

VENTRICULAR TACHYCARDIA. The development of ventricular tachycardia in a patient sustaining an acute myocardial infarction is an ominous sign. This condition frequently and rapidly deteriorates into a more lethal arrhythmia of ventricular fibrillation or asystole.

Ventricular tachycardia may respond to a lidocaine bolus of 50 to 100 mg. If the ventricular tachycardia is not converted with lidocaine, it will be necessary to apply countershock if the patient is unconscious. The monitor defibrillator should be set on the cardioversion mode as opposed to the defibrillation mode.

The lethal arrhythmias of ventricular fibrillation and asystole have already been covered in the section on advanced cardiac life support.

Congestive Heart Failure

Congestive heart failure is a complication that may be seen following the insult of acute myocardial infarction. The initial symptom of support failure may be dyspnea or orthopnea. A sustained sinus tachycardia with a gradual increase in rate may also indicate early congestive heart failure. This is especially true when the pain and anxiety seen with acute myocardial infarction are relieved. Other signs and symptoms are basilar pulmonary rales, a ventricular gallop, and elevation of the central venous pressure, which will be demonstrated by distention of the external jugular neck veins. If the left congestive heart failure is more severe than the right, the patient may present with pink frothy sputum, respiratory distress and expiratory wheezing, cyanosis, sweating, and cold skin. When pink frothy sputum is seen, the patient is headed toward the most severe form of congestive heart failure, pulmonary edema.

Treating the patient with congestive heart failure includes oxygen therapy at 4 to 6 liters per minute, preferably administered by a non-rebreathing mask. The patient, however, usually will not tolerate the mask but will tolerate a cannula. The head of the bed should be elevated, intravenous infusion of D_5W started, and constant cardiac monitoring performed.

Drug therapy is instituted to relieve the venous return to the heart. Morphine sulfate (4 to 8 mg) may be given intravenously to relieve respiratory distress and anxiety and to cause some peripheral vasodilation, thus relieving some of the venous return to the heart. Diuretics such as furosemide may be given intravenously (40 to 80 mg). If the patient is not currently on digitalis, a rapid-acting intravenous form such as Tanatoside C (Cedilanid) may be given in the amount of 0.8 mg.

If pulmonary edema is evident, it may be necessary to apply a rotated tourniquet to trap venous blood in the extremities and thus relieve the workload of the heart.

During transport, attempt to stabilize the patient in preparation for a chest x-ray.

Severe sudden chest pain and syncope suggest acute massive pulmonary embolism. Administer 100 per cent oxygen at a rate of 8 to 10 liters per minute and 5000 units of heparin intravenously to relieve bronchospasm. **Cardiogenic shock** may be present as a result of right ventricular dilation and overload. Isoproterenol, 1 mg in 500 ml of lactated Ringer's solution, is given to produce pulmonary vasodilatation. Atropine may be given, 1.0 mg intravenously, in the treatment of significant bradyarrhythmia. Central venous pressure, arterial blood gases, CBC, and serum enzyme levels should be evaluated as soon as possible.

p. 32

BLUNT AND PENETRATING INJURIES

Following any type of cardiac trauma, the primary concern is resuscitation including the establishment of an adequate airway. A rapid estimation of the extent of a thoracic injury is completed by auscultation of the lungs, observation of movements of the uncovered chest, palpation of the cardiac impulse, and examination of the peripheral pulses with particular attention to the carotid and femoral arteries and the arteries of the extremities. Physical examination may detect subcutaneous emphysema, distention of neck veins, and displacement of the trachea.

Blunt Trauma to the Heart

Myocardial damage following blunt trauma can vary from a small area of hemorrhage to rupture. Myocardial contusion can produce a spectrum of findings ranging from cardiac irritability (manifested by premature contractions) to myocardial infarction. This kind of injury should be suspected in any patient involved in a head-on collision, particularly with steering column or dashboard damage.

Cardiac Tamponade

Cardiac tamponade usually results from penetrating injuries of the heart. Blood fills the pericardial sac and cannot escape. The increased pressure within the pericardial space primarily affects diastolic filling of the heart. Systolic myocardial contraction is rarely limited; however, there is decreased cardiac output as a result of failure of the heart to fill adequately. In acute injuries as little as 150 to 250 ml of blood may be sufficient to cause tamponade, in contrast to the patient with chronic pericardial effusion, in whom tamponade requires as much as a liter of fluid. Shock is clinically evident with cool moist skin, distant heart sounds, and rapid pulse. The jugular veins and veins of the face are distended, and there is cyanosis. A decrease in urinary output may occur.

Treatment

Pre-hospital management of pericardial tamponade at the EMT-A level requires rapid transport to the hospital. This is one of the few emergencies that should be transported using red light and siren.

Close attention should be directed to not overloading the patient with fluid. The distinction between pericardial tamponade and tension pneumothorax is frequently difficult to make without the assistance of a radiograph. The EMT should closely observe the patient and alert the physician at the hospital that pericardial tamponade is suspected.

At the EMT-Paramedic level, the pericardial tamponade, after diagnosis and consultation with the base hospital physician, can be aspirated. Aspiration can be accomplished utilizing the intercardiac needle for epinephrine injection by simply totally evacuating the preloaded syringe. The approach is subxiphoid, aiming at the left scapula just as with any intracardiac injection. The difference is in the forward advancement of the needle. Forward advancement of the needle should be stopped just after entering the pericardial sac, before moving into the ventricle (Fig. 5–3). Identification of the exact location of the tip of the needle can be enhanced by attaching the V lead of the electrocardiograph to the steel shaft of the needle with an alligator clip. As the needle is advanced a current of injury is immediately identified as the tip of the needle touches the myocardium. Backing off slightly into the pericardial sac, the EMT can then aspirate blood without injuring the myocardium.

One hundred and fifty to 250 ml of blood in the pericardial sac is enough to produce a severe tamponade. Removing a few milliliters may be enough to relieve the pressure, allowing the patient's cardiac output to increase, his distal blood pressure to increase, and his right-sided pressure to decrease. Such a maneuver (removing up to 50 to 75 ml of blood) is life saving in a

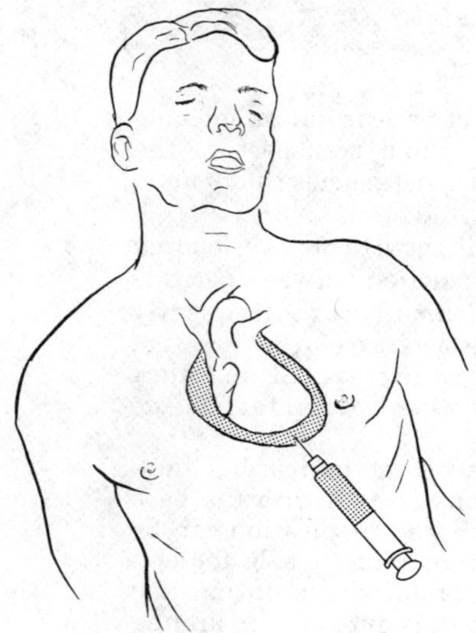

Figure 5–3 Treatment of cardiac tamponade by pericardiocentesis.

severe tamponade situation. It must be kept in mind that this treatment is not definitive but is only a temporizing measure until the patient can be taken to the operating room where, under local anesthesia, a formal pericardiotomy can be accomplished prior to definitive management of the cardiac problem.

Injuries to the cardiac vessels and other interthoracic vascular structures are managed in the pre-hospital period as any other hemorrhagic shock would be with anti-shock trousers and IV infusions.

abdominal and pelvic emergencies

Damage to abdominal and pelvic organs may be caused by penetrating trauma, usually the result of stabs or gunshots, or blunt trauma, resulting from automobile accidents, direct blows, or falls. Although the type and size of the missile and the severity of the impact are usually reflected in the degree of visceral damage, so many variations occur that clinical speculation is dangerous. Wounds that appear to be relatively minor may produce life-threatening internal injuries.

PRINCIPLES

The following principles are the keystones of emergency medical care:

1. When internal injury is in doubt, frequent repeated examinations are essential to early diagnosis.

2. Injuries that interfere with breathing or that cause exsanguinating hemorrhage take precedence over abdominal injuries in treatment.

3. Head injuries are especially difficult to assess, and shock should never be attributed to cerebral damage; peritoneal lavage has its greatest value in these patients.

4. Certain constellations of injuries are common, such as fractures of the ribs on the left with splenic injury; pelvic fractures and bladder rupture; and fractures to lumbar pedicles and intestinal transection in seat belt injuries.

5. The diaphragm extends to the fourth intercostal space, and injuries that on superficial examination appear to be limited to the thorax may have diaphragmatic and abdominal components.

6. The pathway of intraabdominal missiles cannot be predicted from the sites of the entrance and exit wounds; these vary with the position of the patient at the moment of injury and with possible deflections of the missile.

7. With penetrating wounds, the patient's back and anal region must be examined as carefully as the flanks and ventral surface.

8. Seat belts may cause complete transection of the intestine with only minimal early clinical signs.

9. The administration of narcotics should be avoided until a definitive decision about the need for surgery has been made because narcotics may obscure clinical findings.

BLUNT ABDOMINAL INJURIES

It is important for those at the scene of a vehicular accident to observe the direction of impact, the condition of the car, where the occupant was seated, and how the seat belt was applied. These facts will help the examiner in determining potential organ damage. If the seat belt was worn loosely and was riding high off the pelvis, there is a greater chance of serious intraperitoneal injury. If the driver's epigastrium was hit by the steering column, retroperitoneal rupture of the duodenum or traumatic pancreatitis could result.

In auto-pedestrian accidents, the most common intraabdominal injuries in order of frequency are those to the liver, spleen, and small and large bowels. There is greater than a 50 per cent incidence of associated head injury.

There is a high incidence of intraabdominal injuries in abused children and beating victims. Two frequent injuries in these cases are a ruptured duodenum and a torn small bowel mesentery.

The most common injuries in falls are those to the liver and spleen, small intestinal tears at the site of mesenteric attachments (ligament of Treitz and ileocecal junction), and tears of the small bowel mesentery.

Initial Management

Shock due to blood loss continues to be the greatest cause of death in abdominal trauma. Lactated Ringer's solution (1000/ml/hr) should be started at the scene of the accident if shock is present or if intraabdominal bleeding is suspected.

p. 35 An **anti-shock garment** is an important addition to the field armamentarium. When acute massive intra-abdominal hemorrhage with shock is present, the use of the garment can save lives. It is important to remember that if the garment is removed before the patient is in the operating room, as much as 2000 ml of fluid will be required to attain the same blood pressure that was present prior to removal.

Diagnosis

The signs and symptoms of serious injury are frequently vague, absent, or late in presenting. Abdominal pain is most frequently present, but guarding of abdominal muscles may often be absent. The blood pressure, even with severe bleeding, may be normal. Pulse rate and bowel sounds are unreliable clues. Examination of the abdominal wall for abrasions, contusions, and tire marks is of some help in raising the suspicion of potential organ involvement.

Since head injuries are frequently associated with abdominal trauma along with the effects of intoxication or drug abuse, neurological signs may not be obtainable or reliable.

If traumatic pancreatitis is suspected, a serum amylase determination will help confirm the diagnosis and should be obtained in the emergency department as part of the diagnostic studies in patients with abdominal injury.

A urinalysis will aid in diagnosing injuries to the bladder and kidneys. If a patient with an abdominal injury is unable to void after reaching the emergency department, a catheter should be inserted into the urinary bladder, a urine specimen obtained for evaluation, and the catheter left in place until the need for further diagnostic studies or treatment has been resolved.

Radiographic studies are usually indicated in patients with abdominal injuries. Such studies should include a chest film, AP and lateral films of the abdomen, cystograms, and pyelograms when indicated.

PENETRATING ABDOMINAL INJURIES

All patients with stab, gunshot, or other potentially penetrating injuries to the abdomen should be initially treated for actual or potential shock (see treatment for blunt injuries) and transported as rapidly as possible to a facility where definitive care can be given.

NONTRAUMATIC ABDOMINAL EMERGENCIES

It is important to be able to distinguish upper gastrointestinal bleeding and intestinal obstruction, which are true emergencies, from other nontraumatic conditions affecting the abdomen. Important signs and symptoms of gastrointestinal bleeding and intestinal obstruction are bleeding, pain, and abdominal distention.

Gastrointestinal Bleeding

If a patient vomits blood, the source of the injury is in the upper part of the gastrointestinal tract — the esophagus, stomach, or duodenum. Vomiting bright red blood is associated with bleeding esophageal varices, which are enlarged veins. This condition occurs as a complication of severe liver disease, as in chronic alcoholism. Support the patient's circulation with blood or lactated Ringer's solution and oxygen; give nothing by mouth.

Vomiting of bright red blood with a history of black stools suggests a bleeding ulcer, which is not as urgent a problem as bleeding esophageal varices. Passage of bright blood in the stool or after a bowel movement is a sign of lower gastrointestinal bleeding from hemorrhoids, diverticula, malignant disease, or polyps. Lower gastrointestinal bleeding is seldom an emergency.

Abdominal Pain

The type, intensity, and history of the pain are important in making a diagnosis. Persistent colicky pain not relieved in any position suggests kidney or biliary stones. Abdominal pain partially relieved by flexing the abdomen and accompanied by distention and fever is most likely caused by pancreatitis, often seen in alcoholics. Severe upper abdominal pain that is aggravated by movement suggests a perforated duodenal ulcer. Sharp pain around the umbilicus, later shifting to the lower right quadrant, suggests appendicitis. Crampy, intermittent pain with vomiting and abdominal distention may be due to intestinal obstruction.

Strangulation of the bowel with interruption of its blood supply produces hypovolemic shock, and the patient should be treated for shock whenever intestinal obstruction is suspected.

Abdominal Mass

A mildly painful or painless pulsating abdominal mass, palpable between the xiphoid process and the umbilicus, sometimes accompanied by back or flank pain radiating into the groin, may be due to a ruptured or leaking abdominal aortic aneurysm. Some patients will have mild or profound shock and hypotension, and they should be treated for shock. A ruptured aneurysm is a surgical emergency, and large intravenous catheters will be needed in the upper extremities to allow for the rapid infusion of blood and fluids during surgery.

PELVIC TRAUMA

Injuries to the pelvis and pelvic organs occur from accidents that cause injury to the abdomen and its contents. A pelvic fracture should be suspected in patients involved in vehicular accidents (automobile, planes, farm equipment, and so on) as well as falls from buildings. Large amounts of blood can be lost in pelvic fractures. Patients will complain of pain in the groin, especially when they move their legs.

When pelvic injury is suspected following a fall or a vehicular accident and there are signs of impending shock intravenous lactated Ringer's solution should be started (1000/ml/hr), and, if the blood pressure is not monitored, the use of an anti-shock garment should be considered.

If a bladder or urethral injury is suspected, a retrograde urethrogram and cystogram may be necessary. When renal injury is a possibility, infusion pyelography may be indicated as well as retrograde pyelography in ureteral injuries. These are specialized techniques requiring trained personnel for performance and interpretation.

When the possibility of these injuries exists, the patient should be transported to a facility where diagnosis confirmation and personnel for appropriate treatment are available.

External genitalia may be injured in many types of accidents and in criminal assault. If lacerations are present, bleeding may be controlled by digital pressure (especially on the prominent vein of the penis) and pressure from a sanitary dressing. It is very important not to pack anything into the vagina in an attempt to stop hemorrhage. A foreign body impaled in the genitalia or inserted into the penis or vagina must be kept in place until it can be removed by a physician.

NONTRAUMATIC PELVIC EMERGENCIES

The abrupt onset of gross hematuria, painful urination, or severe pain in the pelvic region may suggest a number of problems such as urinary tract infection or obstruction, hydronephrosis, and (in men) prostatitis or benign prostatic hypertrophy. None of these conditions is an emergency. However, particularly in adolescent boys, nontraumatic torsion of the testicle or spermatic cord requires early surgical correction to prevent gangrene. This condition is marked by excruciating and at times disabling pain of sudden onset; it is seen less commonly in males after puberty.

The possibility of pregnancy is a primary consideration in the diagnosis of pelvic pain in women of childbearing age (see Chapter 11).

RAPE

Rape is criminal, forcible sexual intercourse with an unconsenting woman or girl. Since there must be medical evidence of intercourse, an accurate history and physical examination are essential to obtain the proper information that the physician will need later in court. State laws vary with respect to procedures to be followed in examination and collection of specimens from the rape victim. Males (men and boys) may also be subject to rape (forcible sodomy).

facial and neck injuries

Any injury above the clavicle secondary to blunt trauma, regardless of severity, indicates a cervical spine fracture until otherwise proven by x-ray. Physical examination cannot rule out fractures; it can only rule out neurological damage.

PRIMARY MANAGEMENT

Management of *airway* problems involving either the oronasal or oropharyngeal passageway and inadequate lung expansion are discussed in Chapter 3.

Hemorrhage is controlled either by direct pressure or by packing the wound with sterile gauze, if available, and applying enough pressure to stop the blood flow. Dry 4 × 4 bandages may be used as packing, and gentle pressure will allow clots to form on the gauze. If greater pressure is necessary, which is frequently the case, it must be directed so that underlying tissues are not further injured. For example, too much pressure on a scalp injury with a skull fracture beneath it could produce brain damage by forcing unstable skull fragments into the brain tissue.

SECONDARY SURVEY

The secondary survey begins at the scalp and proceeds in an orderly manner to the supraclavicular notch, utilizing the look, listen, and feel approach. Examine the scalp from front to back and from one side to the other for lacerations, avulsions, hematomas, and indentations. Any of these might indicate bony damage, which will be revealed by gentle palpation while watching for changes in the patient's facial expression and listening for verbal acknowledgment that the examination produces pain. The entire surface of the face and neck is thus evaluated.

SPECIFIC INJURIES

Eyes

Examine the eyes carefully for foreign bodies beneath the eyelids including dirt, glass, and other material. Look for the presence of contact lenses. If foreign bodies are present, careful bandaging prevents opening of the eyelids until an ophthalmological examination is performed. If extensive debris or chemical material is present, irrigate the eyes with copious amounts of warm saline as soon as possible. The eyes must be carefully evaluated and managed to prevent increasing the damage. A laceration of the globe allowing extravasation of the vitreous (aqueous) humor is made worse by applying pressure to the eyelid. The same is true of a foreign body beneath the lid.

The upper lid is opened by inverting the lid, the lower by pulling downward on it (Fig. 7–1). Pressure should never be placed directly on the eyelid itself. In the absence of foreign bodies or evidence of corneal damage, gentle palpation determines the ocular tension. If softness of the globe is present, indicating the loss of vitreous or aqueous humor, both eyes should be bandaged. Further examination is carried out at the hospital.

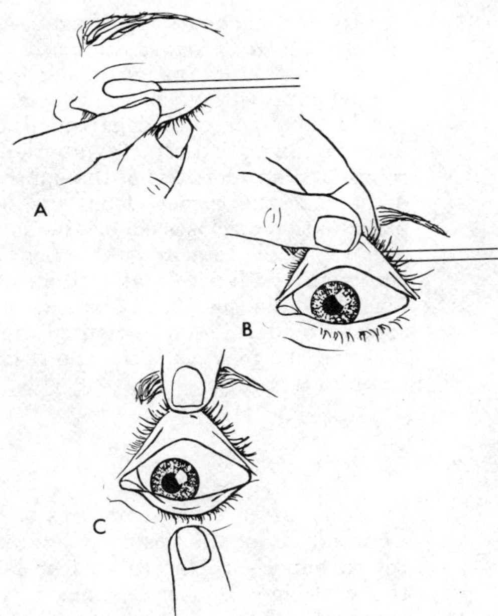

Figure 7–1 *A* and *B*, Retraction of the upper eyelid using a cotton tipped applicator. *C*, Examination of the eye with both lids retracted.

Retraction of the lids permits investigation of the cornea, pupils, conjunctiva, and lenses for damage (loss of both integrity and function). Evaluation of the function of the eyes at this point should always include a test of vision, each eye individually and then both eyes together. The EMT may ask the patient to read some bit of material, such as the lettering on an IV fluid bag. Vision in each eye may be tested at the hospital by using a Snellen eye chart. Diplopia or blurring of vision indicates either dysfunction of the ocular muscles due to nerve damage or entrapment or a blowout orbital fracture. Diplopia can be demonstrated by asking the patient to identify a single object such as a pencil held vertically about 30 cm in front of the nose.

During the neurological evaluation, remember that *eye injuries can produce confusing data*. Injuries to the optic nerve or to the globe itself may cause a fixed, dilated pupil without actual intracranial damage.

In the emergency department, examination should include ophthalmoscopic evaluation utilizing both the round and slit portions of the ophthalmoscope to detect damage to the cornea, lens, and fundus. Funduscopic examination discloses edema, hemorrhage of the retina, and areas of detachment, which is not an unusual occurrence with deceleration injuries. Dislocation of the lens should be specifically looked for, as this itself is an injury. In addition, movement of the lens into an abnormal position may confound the results of a funduscopic examination.

Ears

The ears are frequent sites of laceration. Detailed examination of the posterior and anterior aspects will reveal superficial lacerations or lacerations involving the cartilage. If there is blood emanating from the external auditory meatus, its source must be identified. Clear cerebrospinal fluid may indicate cord damage. A simple laceration causing blood loss does not present with blood coming from behind the tympanic membrane. However, if the tympanic membrane is intact and there is internal bleeding, the blood may not be able to escape to the outside. Therefore, close otoscopic evaluation of the membrane is necessary.

Facial Fractures

Palpation of the zygomatic arches, nasal bones, mandible, and maxilla discloses asymmetry, pain, crepitation, or looseness. Malocclusion of the teeth suggests either fracture of the alveolar ridge or the mandible or dislocations of the temporomandibular joint (Fig. 7-2).

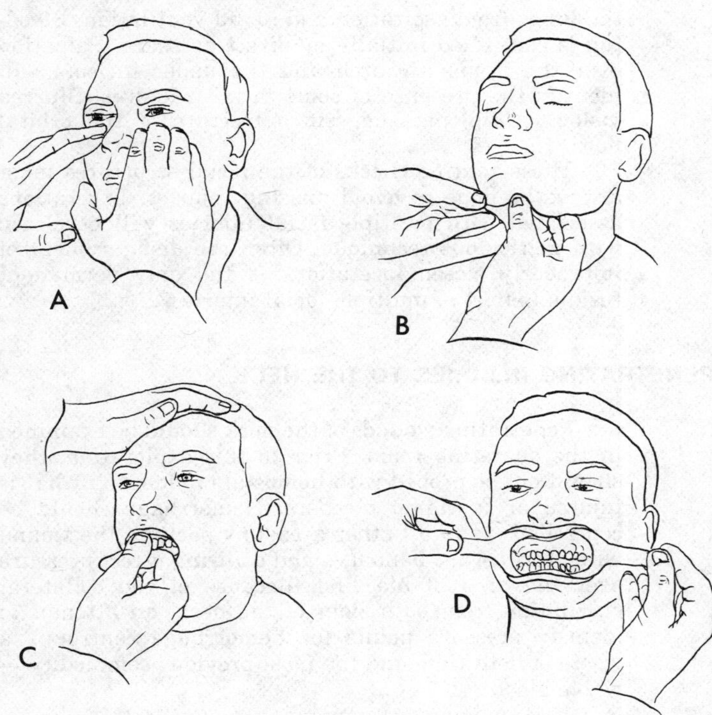

Figure 7–2 *A* and *B*, Palpation of the facial bones. *C*, Attempted manipulation of the maxilla. *D*, Examination of the occlusion.

Multiple Injuries of the Face

It is important to establish priorities when assessing multiple injuries of the face; always evaluate the airway first. Remember that any injury above the clavicle may cause injury to the cervical spine. Because bleeding is commonly associated with multiple facial injuries, a nasal endotracheal tube is frequently required to protect the lungs from aspiration and to aid ventilation. Bleeding is controlled initially by direct pressure. Palpation over the zygomatic arch and the upper incisors will identify the presence of some facial fractures. Blurred vision or diplopia suggests a fracture of the orbital floor.

These routine checks of the facial structures must always be done to avoid missing injuries. Lacerations associated with multiple facial injuries will be closed with meticulous technique. Often the disfigurement of improperly closed lacerations is the only permanent residual effect of multiple facial injuries.

PENETRATING INJURIES TO THE NECK

Penetrating wounds of the neck should be examined in the operating room. Prior to this exploration, they should not be probed with hemostats to identify what is injured or to clamp bleeders. Hemorrhage should be controlled (as in all other areas) by packing the wound with sterile 4× 4 bandages and utilizing direct pressure over the area of bleeding. Because of the collateral circulation from both sides of the neck, an attempt to identify pressure points for hemorrhage control is a waste of both time and the most previous commodity — whole blood.

CERVICAL FRACTURES

Cervical fractures commonly occur when the cervical spine has to absorb the energy of deceleration of the trunk. The cervical spine is treated in the same manner as a cervical fracture in any patient who has received blunt trauma and who has an obvious injury to the clavicle and above, even if the injury is as simple as a laceration or an abrasion on the head.

It is not enough to examine a patient and assume that there is no cervical spine damage because no neurological deficit is present. *Absence of neurological deficits means absence of cord damage, not absence of fractures.*

An unstable fracture without cord damage can cause motor and sensory loss. These nerve injuries are, in general, irreversible, and great care must be taken to prevent their occurrence by proper stabilization of the fracture.

The **extrication technique** is important, as is immobilization of the cervical spine with a short backboard and cervical collar. In the emergency department, continued protection of the cervical spine is absolutely necessary until a lateral x-ray view of the spine visualizing all seven cervical vertebrae rules out the possibility of fracture. Palpation of the cervical spine can frequently identify fractures or dislocations, but only x-ray can rule them out.

p. 186

cerebrospinal injuries

Anyone rendered unconscious as a result of a vehicular crash or a fall must be considered to have *both* head and spine injuries. Brain injury accounts for many deaths following trauma, and serious brain damage that is not lethal causes invalidism in many accident victims. Adequate early emergency medical care can help reduce fatalities and serious, irreversible damage in many of these victims.

It is important for the emergency department physician to know the magnitude of the force that caused the injury. For example, passengers in small cars are often more seriously injured in collisions than similarly placed passengers in heavy cars. A head-on collision is more likely to cause serious injury to the driver of a rear-engine vehicle than to the driver of a front-engine car. An accident causes more trauma at high speeds than at low speeds. In addition, it must be stressed that apparently minor injuries, especially in children, can be lethal. The metal axle of a plastic toy car hurled by a rotary lawnmower against the side of a child's head can cause major problems.

Another important point in the history of the injury is the direction of the traumatic force. A heavy object dropped directly on the head may cause a skull fracture, a compression fracture of the cervical vertebrae, or both. Injuries to the front of the head can cause extreme hyperextension of the neck and can produce a cervical spine fracture or dislocation with or without quadriplegia, yet the brain may be spared.

Seat belts and shoulder harnesses, although added safety features, may spare the brain but can cause spine injuries with or without para- or quadriplegia. A victim propelled from, or a pedestrian struck by, a vehicle is likely to sustain greater injury than a person found injured inside the vehicle. The ambulance staff should obtain this type of information unless emergency treatment of life-threatening injuries precludes taking the necessary time. The information should be relayed to the emergency department physician.

NEUROLOGICAL EXAMINATION

A quick neurological examination should be performed on every patient who has some obvious form of central nervous system dysfunction. However, the general condition of the patient must be evaluated first, searching for airway problems, active external bleeding, signs of shock, and extremity fractures. When the airway is deemed to be adequate, bleeding and shock are under control, fractures are splinted, and vital signs are recorded, one concentrates on the nervous system.

The neurological examination should be simple. If the patient can talk and/or follow a command, he is considered conscious, and this should be recorded. If he does neither, he is unconscious and his response to a painful stimulus should be described as appropriate, feeble, or none. Pupillary size and equality as well as a simple description of extremity strength (strong, weak, or none) should be recorded.

INJURIES TO THE BRAIN

Intracranial injuries include concussion, contusion, laceration, and hemorrhage. *Concussion* is a reversible injury. The patient may be unconscious for anywhere from a few seconds to a few minutes. The more severe the concussion, the more likely it is that the patient will not remember the accident or a period of time afterward (amnesia). In fact, the victim may not recall the accident or a period of time before the injury (retrograde amnesia). Slurred speech is not uncommon in concussion. If the occipital lobe is concussed, temporary visual loss can occur. Staggering or incoordination can result from concussion of the cerebellum. These symptoms usually disappear within hours.

If the brain is *contused*, neurological dysfunction depends on the locale and severity of the contusion. Recovery is slow and often incomplete. Brain *laceration* frequently results in continued bleeding within the brain, which further enlarges the laceration. This is in contrast to a subdural or epidural *hemorrhage*, which compresses the brain as the bleeding continues.

When the brain is injured, fluid tends to collect at the site (cerebral edema). It has been said that cerebral edema kills more people than do blood clots. Except when cerebral edema is most severe, careful patient management can result in survival. Cerebral edema may mimic a blood clot.

The EMT may find a patient uncooperative, agitated, and wishing to be left alone, a typical early finding in a patient who has an enlarging intracranial blood clot. The appearance of hysteria is more likely to be an emotional response to the injury rather than an indication of significant brain damage or intracranial bleeding. Patients who are combatant are likely to be under the influence of drugs or alcohol. Many adults who are involved in vehicular accidents have recently ingested alcoholic beverages, and the odor will be obvious. Nevertheless, these types of behaviors must be considered to be organically based until proved otherwise. *Never consider a patient to be drunk when a head injury has occurred.*

MANAGEMENT

Every unconscious patient must be considered to have an inadequate airway. If he is on his back, secretions or vomitus can flow into the trachea and cause pulmonary complications. The jaw relaxes and the tongue falls backward, adding to upper airway obstruction. Usually if the jaw is elevated and brought forward, this relieves the upper airway obstruction. However, the patient is still unable to handle his secretions adequately owing to a decreased cough reflex.

Unconscious persons who have been involved in a vehicular accident or a fall must always be considered to have a cervical spine injury, and the airway must be managed accordingly. If the airway is compromised, the possibility of a spinal injury is of secondary consideration, especially if the patient is not breathing. Turning the patient three-quarters face down — in a semi-prone position — and maintaining the head in a neutral position during the turn is a good method for relieving partial airway obstruction (Fig. 8–1). In such a position vomitus and secretions tend to run out of the mouth and not down the trachea. The tongue, by gravity, tends to be pulled away from the posterior pharyngeal wall. Other methods to ensure an adequate **airway** are discussed in Chapter 3. p. 11

Any patient who has sustained a head injury may develop *convulsions* at the scene or en route to the hospital. Convulsions are a serious complication of head injuries because of further compromise of the airway. Naturally, when the limbs are forcefully moving in a convulsion, co-existing fractures may produce further damage or bleeding at the fracture site. During a convulsion, maintenance of the airway is difficult but is usually aided by the semi-prone position. If possible, a padded bite-board should be inserted between the teeth to keep the mouth open. The bite-board also prevents damage to the tongue and inside of the mouth due to jaw movement.

Anti-convulsant medications are dangerous and should be administered only by persons trained in their

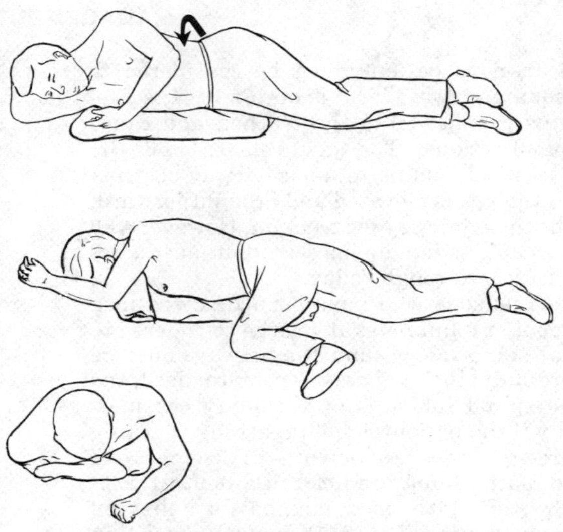

Figure 8–1 Relieving partial airway obstruction in unconscious accident victim with possible spinal injury.

use. To stop a convulsion in a 70-kg adult, 10 mg of diazepam (Valium) can be administered over a two-minute period. This fast-acting drug usually stops the seizure, but its administration should not be repeated. After the seizure stops it may be advisable to give intravenous phenytoin (Dilantin), 50 mg/ml, either prophylactically or to supplement the diazepam. Phenytoin must be given either directly into the vein or with tubing. The dosage is 15 mg per kilogram of body weight; for the average size person, give 1 gm intravenously (at the rate of 50 mg/min). Smaller persons would get less; larger persons would get more. The pulse should be monitored during phenytoin administration in the elderly and in those with heart disease.

Vomiting can occur in any patient with a head injury, especially in a person who is developing an epidural hemorrhage. It can occur even if the patient is unconscious, and this is another reason for the semi-prone position. Catheter aspiration of the upper airway frequently provokes vomiting.

Unconscious patients have difficulty tolerating *temperature* extremes. In contradistinction to patients with spinal cord injuries, the patient with a head injury tends to develop a high temperature. Blankets should not be used if the air temperature is 70° F or above.

With an *open fracture* of the skull, brain tissue commonly oozes out — at times it may even resemble toothpaste. Extrusion of the brain may be beneficial by reducing intracranial pressure. No harm is done to the relatively silent part of the nervous system; later, neuro-surgical repair will be required. A protective sterile dressing should be loosely applied and not compressed against the brain.

Low blood pressure is rarely the result of brain damage and must be considered to be caused by either spinal cord injury or blood loss. When intravenous fluids are administered in the field there is always a tendency for large volumes to be given over a short period of time. This can be very dangerous in the patient with a brain injury because cerebral edema will occur, increasing intracranial pressure. If shock is present, however, the use of intravenous fluids depends on the protocol for shock, not for brain injury. Otherwise, fluids should be administered no faster than 1 ml per minute to keep the intravenous line open for medications.

Cerebrospinal fluid running from either the nose or the ear requires no treatment in the early phase of head injury management. Neither the nose nor the ear should be packed to prevent the fluid from escaping. A loose dressing may be applied to prevent contamination. However, it should be noted on the ambulance and emergency department records that a leak was observed, for it may stop before the patient arrives at the emergency department.

A person who is shocked by high voltage wires may sustain a head injury due to the fall, and the **electrical shock** may injure the spinal cord, the brain, or both.

p. 155

Convulsions are common. It is rare for electrical shock to cause intracranial bleeding requiring emergency surgery.

Scalp bleeding can be severe and can even produce hypovolemic shock. Vigorous bleeding from the scalp can be controlled with simple techniques. Unless a depressed fracture is present, compression by the fingertips against the edge of the wound will stop most bleeding. Pressure over the principal scalp arteries can be effective in temporarily reducing bleeding. Compression dressings usually reduce active bleeding to a slight ooze.

When these simple measures fail or are impractical, as with a depressed skull fracture, hemostats can be applied. Since most of the scalp vessels are small, thin, and numerous, it is impossible to clamp each one. Furthermore, hemostats will fail to hold since the tissue is frail. Instead, the galea, the thin whitish tissue just below the fatty layer of the scalp, is clamped with the tip of the hemostat and the handle deflected away from the laceration. Hemostats are applied every 2 to 3 cm, depending on the size of the wound. There is little pain when the galea is clamped. Self-retaining retractors can be used in the unconscious patient to spread the wound taut until the bleeding stops. After the hemostats or self-retaining retractors are used, the wound is gently packed with sterile gauze and then covered with a bandage.

In rare cases vigorous bleeding continues until the wound is packed. This suggests that the source is not the scalp but either the dural blood vessels or the brain itself. Since packing the wound prevents the blood from escaping, the brain becomes compressed and neurological deterioration follows. One is left with the dilemma of seeing a patient die from either hemorrhage or brain compression. In this situation the dressing can be removed periodically to allow the blood to escape. This decompresses the brain and the patient improves. After the packing has been reapplied, the patient is treated for blood loss. This intermittent application of dressing decreases the amount of bleeding during transport yet prevents death due to brain compression.

SPINAL CORD INJURY

Any of the following findings in an unconscious patient strongly suggests spinal cord injury:

1. The patient has been in a vehicular accident, has fallen a distance, or has an injury above the clavicle;

2. The limbs are flaccid with no tone or reaction to painful stimuli;

3. Chest movement with respiration is feeble; cervical injury should be suspected if the neck muscles contract on inspiration;

4. There are facial grimaces when a painful stimulus is applied above the clavicle but not when applied below the nipples;

5. There is hypotension without obvious blood loss or other evidence of shock; or

6. There is penile erection in the male.

Clinical Syndromes

Spinal cord syndromes often result in peculiar sensations (paresthesias), especially when the skin is touched. This sensation may be no more than the feeling of "pins and needles," or it may be extremely disagreeable.

When spinal cord injury is incomplete, symptoms are variable. There may be weakness or paralysis, which may be asymmetrical, with sensation remaining normal. The patient may complain only of paresthesia. Lesions in the neck or lumbar area can produce a confused picture. In the case of a lesion at the sixth cervical vertebra, the forearms may be flexed across the chest, since the biceps can contract but the triceps cannot. A lesion at the first lumbar level may produce sensory loss below the top of an imaginary bikini. With a lesion at the third lumbar level, hip flexion is good, but the patient may not be able to move his feet or toes.

Uncommonly, cord concussion can occur, with complete and rapid recovery. Cord injury usually results in some permanent loss, and not infrequently no recovery occurs. Spinal cord injury that produces a total loss of neural function is known as spinal shock. The patient cannot move his limbs. There is no reflex action and sensation is gone. The blood pressure is low and there may be a slow or normal pulse rate. If the lesion is in the lower cervical region, the intercostal muscles are paralyzed, so that breathing is performed by the diaphragm. Urinary bladder and rectal functions are lost. The male may have an erection. Sweating and shivering capabilities may be absent, which interferes with temperature regulation.

If spinal shock occurs above the fourth cervical vertebra, the diaphragm is also paralyzed. Such paralysis may not cause immediate death, because the neck muscles and the contractions of the heart may be able to produce enough respiratory exchange to keep the heart and brain working for a time. However, this marginal breathing soon produces cerebral anoxia with unconsciousness and, usually, dilated fixed pupils. Cerebral anoxia often mimics head injuries. Respiratory resuscitation can reverse cerebral anoxia, but the patient will require a respirator unless cord concussion was the cause of the spinal shock.

Hemisection of the spinal cord, which occurs primarily with knife or ice pick injuries, produces an ipsilateral paralysis below the level of the injury with position sense impairment on the same side. However, there is loss of pain and temperature senses on the opposite side of the body. Touch is usually not affected.

Damage to the *anterior spinal artery* produces weakness or paralysis of the lower limbs with loss of pain and temperature sensation. Position sense and touch are present. Reflexes may be diminished or increased, and the legs may be flaccid or spastic.

Central cord injury is a spinal cord syndrome that primarily occurs with neck injuries, especially in elderly people with advanced arthritis of the cervical spine. A momentary hyperextension of the neck causes acute compression of the spinal cord, which may never function again. Less commonly, forced flexion can have the same effect, but this is usually associated with fracture of a vertebral body. The hands are numb and motionless, and there is urinary retention. Recovery occurs first in the legs; the hands usually never fully recover.

Another feature of spinal injury is *pain over the spine* at the site of impact. This pain is increased with movement. A nerve root exits on each side between each two vertebral bodies, so there can be pain in the segmental distribution of one or more of the nerve roots (radicular pain). Sometimes the sensation supplied by these roots is perverted, resulting in a very annoying type of sensation when the patient is touched. It must be stressed that spinal cord injuries can present without fracture or pain.

Neurological Examination

One of the indications for neurosurgery is progressive deterioration. Therefore, a baseline examination is important. There is no easy check system for spinal injuries, but a brief description of what the patient can do, such as wiggle the toes or flex the thighs, may be invaluable later. The sensory level should be marked on the skin with ink. For example, if there is loss of sensation below the umbilicus when the patient is first seen and later the level rises to the rib cage, this may be evidence of epidural spinal hemorrhage. As with the brain, rapid surgical decompression is needed. On the other hand, when serial examination indicates improvement, spinal surgery will not be required except to stabilize the spine.

A complete sensory examination requires too much time in emergency situations. However, certain areas should be checked as follows:

1. Top of the little toe (S1)
2. Just above the knee cap (L3)
3. Below the iliac crest (L1)
4. At the level of the umbilicus (T10)
5. At the lower tip of the sternum (T6)
6. At the nipples (T4)
7. Tip of the fifth finger (C8)
8. Tip of the ring finger (C7)

9. Tip of the thumb (C6)
10. Top of the shoulder (C4)
11. Two inches behind the tip of the ear (C2)
12. The skin near the anus, checked by gently lifting the leg.

It is not uncommon for an incomplete lesion to primarily affect the lower limbs but spare the sensory supply around the anus. On the other hand, the anus may be the only site of sensory loss. Therefore, every sensory examination should include the anal area unless fractures prevent movement of the lower limbs.

As with the sensory system, examination of muscle action can produce a confusing picture, depending on the location of the cord injury. With injuries at C4 or above there is paralysis of the respiratory muscles. The victim of an injury at C6 is often found with his hands half open and in the "hold up" position, or the upper limbs may be flexed over the chest, because the biceps or deltoid muscles are functioning but the triceps are paralyzed.

At L3 there is hip flexion and adduction, and at L5 the only extremity weakness may be in the extensor muscles of the foot or toes, so that the patient can flex but cannot extend the foot or great toe.

Often the patient is asked to wiggle his toes and may be able to do so, giving the impression that there is no weakness when the lesion is above L4. In actuality he is able to flex his toes voluntarily, and upon relaxing they come back to a neutral position.

A lesion in the lower cervical vertebrae almost always produces weakness of hand grip. For muscle examination, the biceps is tested to see if the forearm can flex strongly. The triceps is examined by having the patient extend the forearm. In the lower extremity, the ability to flex the thigh against resistance and to dorsiflex the great toe or the foot is important.

Special Problems

Since the diagnosis of fractures or dislocations can be made only by x-ray, every patient suspected of having a spinal fracture should be treated as if the diagnosis had been confirmed. The percentage of cord injuries with fractures is much higher in the cervical area, and the chance for a second accident to occur during movement must be avoided. Following auto accidents, patients suspected of having sustained spine injuries should be removed from the vehicle by applying a *short spine board* whenever possible. Once removed, the patient can be transported on a rigid stretcher or a long spine board with proper immobilization of the head, using sand bags and adhesive tape. Special litters and attachments are available, but short and long spine boards can be made inexpensively and easily from 3/4-in plywood strips.

Airway support may be needed promptly. Intubation is difficult in neck injuries because the cervical spine cannot be hyperextended safely; however, if the patient is in respiratory distress there may be no alternative unless the ambulance personnel have been trained in surgical technique. The **esophageal obturator airway** may have merit in these cases, for this method also prevents vomiting. Vomiting is a likely complication of intubation, especially if the patient has recently eaten or consumed a great deal of fluid. If this is the case and the airway appears adequate, it may be advisable to pass a stomach tube and aspirate the contents. By reducing the size of the stomach, diaphragm action is made more efficient.

p. 18

Part of the picture of spinal shock is hypotension, often with bradycardia. The other clinical features of shock, such as pallor and sweating, are usually absent.

Spinal injury reduces respiratory efficiency; coupled with the expected low blood pressure, this can result in cerebral anoxia. The patient becomes apprehensive and may lapse into a coma and even develop dilated fixed pupils. An intravenous injection of 1% Neo-Synephrine solution can increase the blood pressure and can actually awaken the patient. This is contraindicated if one suspects that the hypotension is due to blood loss.

In the presence of pain or disagreeable paresthesias, the patient may beg for medication. Unfortunately, the type and dosage of medication needed to obtain relief can adversely affect respiration and blood pressure. It may be better to withhold pain medication during transportation. If it is felt to be absolutely necessary, an intravenous injection of diazepam, 10 mg over a two- to five-minute period, may be helpful. It should also be pointed out that in the quadriplegic or paraplegic patient, intramuscular medication may be poorly absorbed.

Urinary bladder paralysis is a frequent finding in spinal injuries. If the estimated time lapse from the accident site to arrival at the hospital is more than four hours, a urinary catheter should be inserted. The patient will have no bladder sensation and does not realize the need to urinate. Overdistention of the bladder must be avoided.

extremity injuries

Injuries to the extremities are seldom a cause of death in trauma patients, so it is not surprising that the establishment and maintenance of a satisfactory airway, proper ventilation, and measures to control bleeding and restore blood loss take precedence over their management. It is important to remember that the consequences of extremity injuries may add to the seriousness of these life-threatening problems in three ways.

1. The pain associated with extremity injuries may contribute to the patient's **shock**. This pain can be largely eliminated with proper splinting and immobilization. p. 32

2. The extremities may be a site of **fluid loss.** Extremity bleeding is often readily controlled by simple measures such as elevation, pressure dressings, and the use of a blood pressure cuff as a tourniquet. The movement of blood and plasma into injured extremities results in considerable swelling. Blood loss must also be considered in plans to restore the patient's blood volume. p. 167

3. The skin covering the four extremities makes up over 50 per cent of the total body surface and when burned, cut, or abraded becomes a potential entry site for **infection**. Early recognition and proper attention to these wounds, including the application of sterile dressing, the judicious use of antibiotics, and proper surgical p. 89

treatment, may prevent the years of disability associated with bone and joint infections or the development of life-threatening infections such as tetanus or gas gangrene.

It is therefore vital to recognize that the proper treatment of the extremity injury is not only essential to the ultimate function of that part but may play a major role in the survival of the patient who has also incurred other injuries.

TYPES OF EXTREMITY INJURIES

As in other body areas, two general categories of injury are encountered in the extremities. *Penetrating injuries* are those in which some object, such as a knife, bullet, piece of glass, or even a splinter of wood, penetrates the skin of the extremity leaving an *entrance wound*. Such wounds are often misleading, since they seldom provide a clue to the magnitude and extent of underlying injury. Since they represent a portal for bacteria, they should be carefully noted and covered with a sterile dressing. If the object that created the wound is still in place, e.g., a knife blade or fence post, it should not be withdrawn but instead should be stabilized and transported with the patient. Bullets that enter extremities may remain within the tissues and will occasionally be felt just beneath the skin. Their location is best confirmed by x-ray studies in two dimensions. In some instances, the missile or knife blade will continue through the tissues and leave a second opening or *exit wound*, which should also be noted and covered by sterile dressing. If bleeding from the exit wound is excessive, pressure should be applied.

The treatment of penetrating wounds of the extremities is based on the extent of injury to the underlying bones, nerves, blood vessels, and muscles. These deeper injuries will be obvious in some instances by the presence of active bleeding or the loss of circulation, sensation, or movement distal to the penetration site. However, assessment of the extent of damage is neither possible nor advisable at the scene of the accident.

Rather, the person providing first aid should assume that concealed injuries are present and should cover the wounds, immobilize the extremity, and arrange for definitive diagnosis and treatment as soon as possible.

The second category of extremity injuries includes those resulting from forces that do not break the skin or that do so only after greatly deforming the extremity. These blunt or *nonpenetrating injuries* are much more frequent than penetrating injuries and include most sprains, dislocations, fractures, and bruises. The injuring force may be externally applied, as when the legs are struck by an automobile bumper; or the injury may result from a twisting motion or misstep (e.g., an ankle fracture or sprain). Such injuries may lead to fractures in which the broken bone actually protrudes through the skin. When this occurs, the same risks of infection arise as with penetrating wounds.

The likelihood of bone and joint injury is increased in nonpenetrating extremity injuries, but the underlying nerves, blood vessels, and muscles may also be injured. Except for obvious deformities or circulation impairment, the extent of underlying injury can usually only be determined after a careful physical examination and x-ray studies. Until these are complete, underlying injury should be assumed and the involved extremity elevated, immobilized, and protected from further injury.

SPECIFIC INJURIES

Skin and Subcutaneous Tissues

Injuries to the skin and subcutaneous tissues may be caused by cold, heat, abrasions, cuts, splinters, needles, missiles, and underlying bones.

Intact and normal skin is a barrier against bacteria, so it is important to preserve and protect it. Once the skin is broken, care and judgment should be exercised in deciding when and how to repair it. The history of the wound and the extent of prior treatment are major considerations in deciding on definitive care. Emergency care consists of controlling hemorrhage and protecting the wound against further contamination. Subsequent treatment involves surgical exploration, debridement, splinting, and closure.

Blood Vessels

The circulation of blood to the extremity is provided by large arteries about a centimeter in diameter that enter at the groin and the axilla. These arteries continue near the bone and separate into smaller branches as they progress to the tips of the fingers and toes. At certain points along their course these branches are close

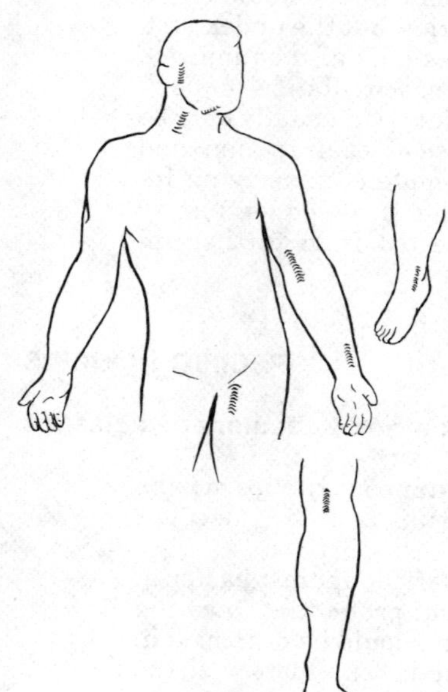

Figure 9–1 Pulse points.

enough to the skin to be felt by the examining finger (Fig. 9–1). These pulse points are useful in establishing the persistence of arterial flow and can occasionally be helpful in controlling bleeding (i.e., the rescuer can apply pressure over an involved artery above the site of injury).

The blood returns to the heart from the extremities by way of a system of veins, which are larger and more numerous than the arteries. The pressure in the veins is low as compared with that in the arteries, and venous bleeding will usually stop quickly in response to mild pressure or elevation (to "empty" blood from the venous system).

External Hemorrhage

Injuries to the arteries or veins of an extremity may lead to the loss of considerable amounts of blood, contributing to the development of shock and even leading to the death of the patient. Fatal blood loss usually occurs only with penetrating wounds or amputations. Major bleeding through a break in the skin is best controlled by the application of direct pressure. If the bleeding continues in spite of direct pressure, it can usually be stopped by applying the pressure a little above or below the skin break. When necessary, an air splint can be applied for more effective pressure. A circular bandage, a blood pressure cuff, or any other tourniquet is to be reserved for hemorrhage uncontrolled by any other method.

Internal Hemorrhage

For most nonpenetrating injuries, the intact skin and surrounding muscles serve as a tourniquet to limit the loss of blood from injured vessels. Considerable amounts of blood may be lost from the circulation into concealed tissues, and such losses must be considered in the resuscitation of injured patients.

Loss of arterial circulation to an extremity may be recognized in several ways.

1. The skin of the involved extremity is seen to be white or blue when compared with the opposite extremity.

2. The skin is cool to the touch.

3. Pulsations are not felt at the usual sites (wrist, ankle, dorsum of the foot).

4. Sensibility to a pin prick is decreased in the distal parts of the extremity.

When any of these changes are noted, the extremity should be checked for a deformity suggestive of fracture or dislocation. Apply traction, and splint and elevate the extremity. Replace the lost blood with intravenous lactated Ringer's solution in large amounts as necessary to maintain blood pressure.

Whether or not the patient responds to these measures, the findings should be recorded and the patient transported promptly to the hospital.

Serious vascular injury may occur without any of the immediate findings previously mentioned. Accurate diagnosis in the hospital often involves the periodic evaluation of pulse and blood pressure in the limb, listening with a stethoscope over the sites of injury, and the use of angiography, particularly in patients with penetrating wounds. What might initially appear to be an intact circulatory system may undergo late obstruction with the characteristic signs of vascular injury presenting hours or even days later.

Nerves

The major sensory and motor nerves of an extremity follow pathways similar to those of the arteries and veins. These nerves may be cut by penetrating objects, or they may be bruised, stretched, or torn. The result may be loss of function, such as the ability to extend the wrist or rotate the thumb, or loss of awareness to a pin prick over one or both sides of several of the fingers or toes.

Asking the conscious patient to move his extremities may not be practical in the face of other injuries, but suspicion of loss of function should always be recorded and confirmed at the earliest convenient time. The loss of nerve function in the extremity may be due to an injury to the brain or spinal cord, requiring special attention to areas other than the injured extremity. If loss of arterial circulation has occurred owing to ischemia, the nerves of the extremity may fail to function, leading to paralysis or loss of sensation.

Muscles and Tendons

The muscles and tendons of an extremity move the various parts of the limb, and it is obvious that injury to these structures may lead to loss of motion of a forearm, leg, foot, hand, or digit. The involved part should be noted, a splint applied to correct any deformity, and the part elevated to minimize swelling. Penetrating injuries of the hand often result in damage to tendons. The wound should be covered with sterile dressings and a surgical consultation arranged.

With tears or ruptures of muscles and tendons, the extremity should be immobilized and elevated until further evaluation is possible. Wounds should be covered with sterile dressings.

Bones and Joints

If the *joint capsule* or *ligaments* are stretched or torn without escape of one of the bony surfaces, the injury is referred to as a *strain* or *sprain*. If the capsule or ligaments are disrupted and a bony surface escapes, it is called a *dislocation*.

Any break in the bone is a *fracture*. Many different types of fractures and dislocations can occur. The most immediate consideration is whether the bone has penetrated the skin. Such a fracture or dislocation is referred to as an *open* (also called *compound*) *fracture* and requires special precautions to prevent infection. Similarly, if a penetrating injury involves a joint or reaches a bone, the risks of infection are increased.

EMERGENCY SPLINTING OF EXTREMITY INJURIES

General Principles

1. Preservation of life takes priority over emergency splinting. Treat asphyxia, control massive hemorrhage, and initiate therapy for shock before splinting. Effective splinting may help to prevent shock.

2. Examine the injured extremity for signs of arterial and nerve injury before searching for a fracture and providing emergency splinting. Feel for a pulse distal to the fracture.

3. "Splint 'em where they lie" to guard against the conversion of a closed fracture to an open fracture and against further soft tissue drainage.

4. For maximum splinting effectiveness, immobilize the joints above and below a fracture.

5. Standard commercial splints should always be available, but if not, splints may be improvised using tree limbs, folded newspapers, or a pinned upturned shirttail (for a sling).

6. Clothing on the injured extremity must be removed.

Objectives

1. Effective splinting, at the scene or in the emergency department, is an important facet in managing fracture and dislocations.

2. Emergency splinting prevents additional soft tissue damage by bone fragments, minimizes pain, and provides comfort during transport.

3. Splinting must not embarrass circulation or produce pressure on nerves or against bony prominences.

TECHNIQUES OF SPLINTING

It is essential to distinguish between (1) splinting applied temporarily for transportation and (2) splinting applied to hold or achieve reduction of a fracture or dislocation and to provide prolonged immobilization. Splints are of two types, coaptation and traction.

Splinting of Open Fractures or Dislocations

The management of open fractures is directed toward healing the open wound without infection and healing the fracture in good position. To accomplish these two objectives, open fractures or dislocations require the application of a sterile dressing over the wound *before* splinting. Putting antiseptic solutions into or around the wound may be hazardous. Protruding fragments of bone should not be replaced in the wound but should merely be covered with the dressing. In emergency splinting, the amount of traction applied should not cause protruding fragments to recede into the wound. Immediate hospitalization is indicated for open fractures and dislocations. Antibiotic therapy and appropriate antitetanus prophylaxis should be initiated promptly.

Fractures or Dislocations of the Upper Extremity

Evaluation of blood circulation to the hand and peripheral nerve supply to the forearm and hand precedes the application of emergency splinting. A pink, warm hand indicates adequate circulation; pallor or cyanosis indicates impaired circulation. A good radial pulse is a favorable sign. A standard test for circulation can be performed by pressing on the end of a fingernail so as to cause blanching of the nail bed. With good circulation, a pink color promptly replaces the blanched area when pressure on the nail is released. With impaired circulation, the pink color either returns slowly or does not return. All that can be done in the field to manage the impaired circulation is to ensure that tight clothing above the site of injury is not the cause and to correct gross deformity at the injury site prior to appropriate splinting. Circulation to the hand should be retested after splinting.

Evaluation of peripheral nerve function is more difficult. The patient should be asked to flex, extend, and spread the fingers and move the thumb in all directions. With fractures of the forearm or hand, pain from the injury may limit such movements. Sensibility in the hand may be tested by a pin prick; testing by mere touch is not adequate. Nothing can be done at the scene for impaired nerve function other than correction of gross deformity.

All information obtained about circulation and nerve function should be recorded and relayed promptly to the treating physician at the hospital.

Shoulder and Arm

The injured extremity is placed in a sling, usually with the elbow at a right angle, and is bound to the chest with a swathe, bandage, or another sling (Fig. 9–2). Such use of the chest wall is an example of coaptation splinting. For fractures of the humeral shaft, the sling should not be applied so as to lift the forearm. When flexing the elbow at a right angle is very painful, the entire extremity may be bandaged to the trunk with the elbow flexed to about 80°.

When the patient holds his arm away from his side a dislocation of the shoulder rather than a fracture should be suspected. Efforts to bring the arm to the side will be quite painful and should be avoided. A pillow or other soft material should be placed to help hold the arm away from the chest, and a bandage should be applied to hold the pillow and the arm in the most comfortable position. When a sling is not available, the patient's shirttail may

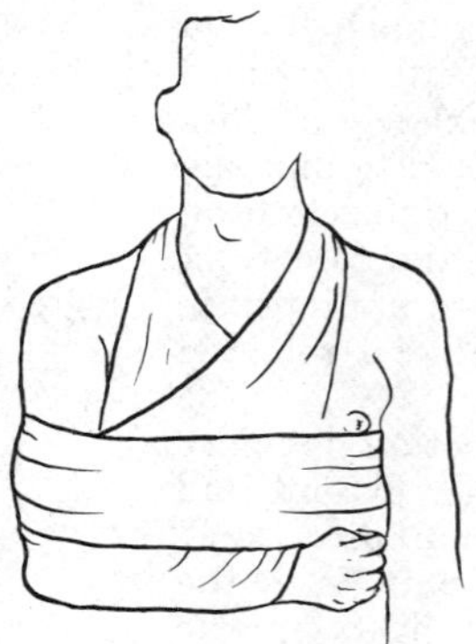

Figure 9–2 Use of a sling and coaptation bandage for fracture of the arm or shoulder.

be turned up and pinned to support the forearm, and the extremity may be bandaged to the chest wall.

Patients with a dislocated shoulder and many patients with a fracture about the shoulder or of the arm will be more comfortable and will transport better in a sitting position.

Elbow

The injured extremity is splinted as found. No attempt should be made to flex the elbow. Coaptation splinting is accomplished by bandaging the entire extremity to the trunk, perhaps after molding a wire ladder splint to the contour assumed by the elbow.

Forearm, Wrist, and Hand

Adequate splinting is seldom a problem with fractures of the forearm, wrist, or hand; coaptation splinting

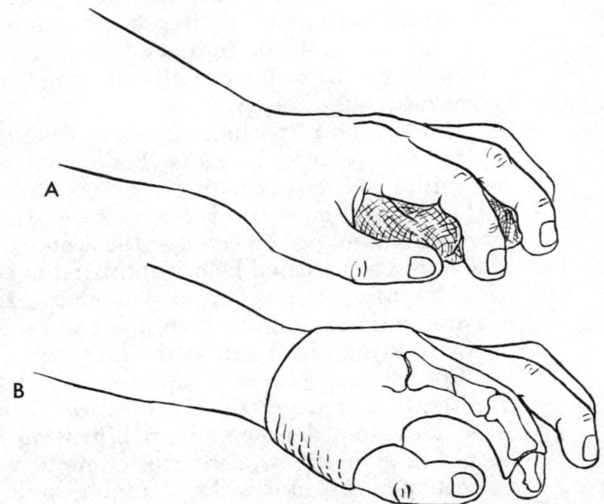

Figure 9–3 Treatment of phalangeal fractures. *A,* Pad the palm with the fingers flexed. *B,* A cast maintains this position.

is used. For fractures near the wrist or of the hand, a padded board is applied to the volar surface; for those of the forearm, boards are used on both front and back. A commercial metal splint or an inflatable air splint is equally effective. For injuries of the hand, padding in the palm is desirable so that the fingers are held in the position of function (Fig. 9-3). A sling holding the elbow at a right angle completes the splinting.

Fractures or Dislocations of the Lower Extremity

Evaluation of the circulation of the foot and of peripheral nerve function in the leg and foot precedes the application of emergency splinting. A pink, warm foot indicates good circulation as do strong pulsations in the posterior tibial and dorsalis pedis arteries. Coolness, pallor, or cyanosis of the foot indicates impaired circulation. Blanching of the toenail beds upon pressure and prompt return of a pink color is a sign of adequate circulation to the foot. If circulation is impaired, ensure that the cause is not tight clothing and correct gross deformity before splinting. Circulation of the foot should be reevaluated after splinting.

Evaluation of peripheral nerve function consists of asking the patient to move his toes and testing for sensibility of the toes with pin pricks. With fractures of the leg, pain may limit toe motion. Impaired nerve function cannot be corrected at the scene. Gross deformity should be corrected before splinting is accomplished.

All information obtained about circulation and nerve function should be recorded and relayed promptly to the treating physician at the hospital.

Splinting fractures or dislocations of the lower extremity is of paramount importance. The patient can often provide a degree of immobilization of an injured shoulder, arm, elbow, forearm, or hand with his uninjured upper extremity. He is unable to do so, however, with complete fractures of the femur or of both bones of the leg. He is usually helpless until aid arrives.

Fractures of the Femur

Traction splinting utilizing a half-ring or full-ring splint is indicated for fractures of the femur. Slings support the extremity in the splint, and traction is applied to an ankle hitch. Loops of bandage, preferably muslin, or folded slings (as used for the upper extremity) tied to the splint uprights may be used to support the extremity. Standard commercial ankle hitches are preferable to improvised hitches made from muslin bandages.

There is one traction splint that offers several advantages (Fig. 9–4). It has supports for the extremity with Velcro grips affixed to the uprights. When the extremity is placed on these supports, the ends are merely folded over it and secured by the grips. The same supplier also offers a broad padded ankle hitch and an adjustable strap that may be passed through the metal loops of the hitch, then looped around the end of the splint and tightened to provide traction.

Applying traction splinting is a two-man process. With the injured extremity free of clothing, the splint placed beside it, and an ankle hitch at hand, one person grasps the ankle and pulls on the extremity; this usually reduces any gross deformity. The second person lifts the injured extremity and slides the splint beneath it. The traction hitch is placed about the ankle and then fixed to the end of the splint with enough tension to provide moderate traction. If the shoe is present, it provides some protection from hitch pressure. The distal end of the traction splint is elevated.

If traction splinting cannot be provided for a fractured femur, coaptation splinting, although less effec-

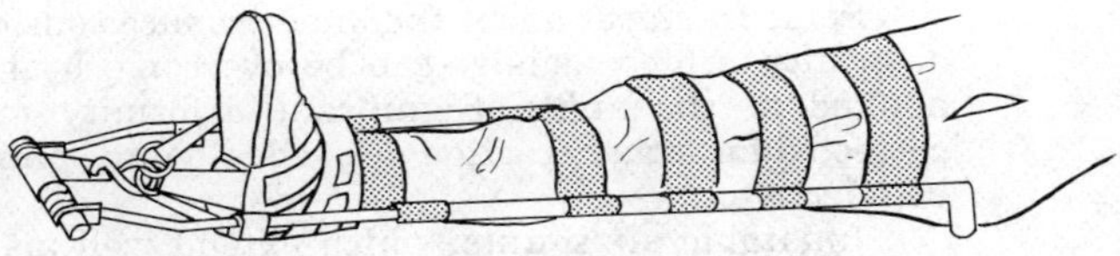

Figure 9–4 A traction splint applied to the lower extremity.

tive, is indicated. While one person provides some traction, another bandages a long padded board splint laterally to the full length of the extremity, extending up along the trunk, including the lower thoracic cage in the absence of associated chest injury. One short padded board is placed medially and another posteriorly.

Inflatable air splints are inadequate for fractures of the femur because the hip joint cannot be included. However, because of the position of anti-shock trousers extending up to the lower lumbar area and down below the knees, fractures of the femur and pelvis can be adequately stabilized. Both the Sagar and Hare traction splints can be applied external to the anti-shock garment, providing inline traction as well as compression immobilization.

Dislocations of the Hip

A dislocated hip joint usually causes the thigh and leg to assume flexed positions. No attempt should be made to reduce this flexion. Supporting pillows or blankets should be placed beneath the thigh and flexed knee and the patient transported to a hospital with the extremity in the position in which it was found.

Fractures about the Knee

Either traction splinting as for fractures of the femur or coaptation splinting using medial and lateral padded boards may be used for fractures about the knee. Traction splinting is preferable for fractures of the distal femur; if board splints are used, the lateral board should extend upward to the pelvic brim. All boards should extend distally beyond the foot.

Some fractures about the knee produce considerable deformity, which usually can be overcome by traction applied at the ankle. Significant deformity must be corrected for either traction or padded board splinting to be effective.

Inflatable air splints, which extend well above the knee, offer effective splinting for fractures of the proximal end of the bones of the lower leg or of the patella, but such splinting is no better than traction or padded board splints for these injuries. Air splints are less than adequate for fractures of the distal end of the femur.

Dislocations of the Knee

The proximal ends of the bones of the leg are usually displaced backward. These dislocations are limb endangering because of a torn or obstructed popliteal artery. Therefore, careful evaluation of the arterial pulsations at the ankle and foot is mandatory. If these pulsations are absent or if the foot shows pallor or cyanosis, a prompt reasonable effort at reduction of the dislocation is indicated. At times, strong, steady, manual traction at the ankle in the long axis of the extremity will effect a complete or partial reduction of the dislocation with complete or partial relief of popliteal artery obstruction. Such an effort is worthwhile at the scene or in the emergency department. The emergency department or hospital physician must be notified promptly about any impaired circulation that was noted.

Splinting for dislocations of the knee, with or without an effort at reduction, is comparable to that described for fractures about the knee. An air splint is unlikely to be adequate for these dislocations.

Fractures of the Leg

For fractures of the shaft of either one or both bones of the leg, coaptation splinting is usually effective, although traction splinting is ideal for those fractures at or near the junction of the proximal and middle thirds of the leg. Coaptation splinting may be provided by an inflatable air splint extending well above the knee; padded board splints placed medially, laterally, and posteriorly, each extending from near the groin to the foot; or a well-padded metal posterior gutter splint. When board splints are used, padding must be arranged so that the malleoli and head of the fibula are protected from painful pressure. Inadequate protection of the head of the fibula can result in excessive pressure on the peroneal nerve, causing paralysis (footdrop).

A pillow splint (a form of improvised coaptation splinting) will provide adequate emergency splinting for fractures of the bones of the leg, particularly in the lower half. The leg is lifted onto a pillow, which is bandaged securely to the leg and lower thigh (Fig. 9–5). Boards placed medially and laterally outside the pillow will enhance the splinting effect. For complete fractures, particularly of both bones, two people are required, one to lift and support the leg, the other to provide splinting.

Inflatable air splints require some precautions during their application. Some are made with a full-length zipper. The leg is placed on the air splint, the zipper is closed, and the splint is inflated by mouth. An air pump should never be used. After inflation, pressure of a thumb or finger should indent the splint slightly without producing detectable pressure on the leg. The amount of inflation should permit the fingers to pass beneath the upper end of the splint with moderate effort. Air splints without a zipper are more difficult to apply. The foot and leg must be fed into the splint.

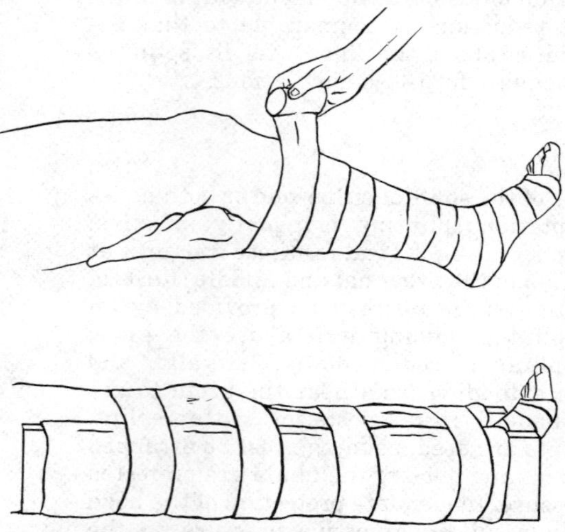

Figure 9–5   A pillow splint applied to the lower extremity.

Fractures about the Ankle

Satisfactory splinting of the ankle is afforded by an air splint, padded boards that extend only to the knee, a well-padded knee-length posterior metal gutter splint, or a pillow splint. When a pillow splint is used, it should be folded and pinned about the foot to obtain maximum immobilization.

Dislocations of the Ankle

Dislocations of the ankle are almost always accompanied by fractures. Gross deformity must be corrected by moderate traction and manipulation before splinting. Any of the splinting methods described for fractures of the ankle are applicable for dislocations.

Fractures or Dislocations of the Foot

Any of the splinting methods mentioned for fractures of the ankle are applicable for fractures or dislocations within the foot. A pillow folded and pinned about the foot is a simple, effective method of splinting these injuries.

special medical emergencies

STATUS EPILEPTICUS

Status epilepticus is a convulsive disorder in which the patient does not regain consciousness between seizures. It most often occurs in patients with known seizure disorders who suddenly discontinue their maintenance therapy.

Although ventilation usually ceases and the patient often becomes cyanotic during a generalized seizure, supplemental oxygen is almost never required. Intubation is rarely needed and should be deferred until the seizure has ceased. An oral airway is suggested to protect the tongue and oral mucosa. A padded tongue blade or folded handkerchief is equally effective.

During a seizure, the patient should be placed in the recumbent position on a flat surface. If the surrounding area can be padded, such as the side rails on a hospital cart or bed, this should be done.

The treatment of choice for status epilepticus is diazepam (Valium), given intravenously in doses up to 10 mg over two minutes. This dosage may be repeated two to four times within an hour. Diazepam must be given slowly, because rapid administration may lead to respiratory arrest. After initial control of the seizure with diazepam, phenytoin (Dilantin) may be given intravenously in doses of 100 to 300 mg, not faster than 100 mg per minute. Phenobarbital (Luminal) can also be given intravenously in doses of 120 to 240 mg at a rate not exceeding 60 mg per minute. The patient should be observed carefully for cardiopulmonary arrest.

ANAPHYLAXIS

Anaphylaxis is an acute systemic reaction by a sensitized person to an antigen. The resultant antigen-antibody reaction can be mild or severe. A mild reaction may consist only of nasal congestion, itching, conjunctivitis, hives, and gastrointestinal symptoms including nausea, vomiting, diarrhea, or abdominal pain. More severe anaphylactic reactions may include laryngeal edema, wheezing, cardiac arrhythmia, hypotension, shock, and even cardiorespiratory arrest. The precipitating antigen may be a drug, contrast medium, venom, or food.

The treatment for anaphylaxis is aqueous epinephrine, 0.3 to 1.0 ml of a 1:1000 solution given subcutaneously or intramuscularly. If the anaphylactic state results from an injection or an insect sting in an extremity, a tourniquet may be applied proximal to the injury site. A patent airway must be maintained. If hypotension is present, the person may respond to the initial dose of epinephrine; however, fluids and vasoconstrictors may be necessary. Aminophylline administered intravenously may be helpful if bronchospasm is present. Oxygen should be administered if the patient is cyanotic or severely dyspneic. Intravenous steroids may be required in severe cases.

POISONING

In cases of ingested poisons, the stomach should be emptied with a large gastric tube. However, gastric lavage should not be attempted after the ingestion of strong acids or alkalis because of the dangers of perforation and further harm to the tissues. Emesis should be induced if the patient is conscious and if the poison is not a caustic or corrosive agent. Emesis can be induced by having the patient drink at least 250 ml of water or milk

and then irritating the posterior pharynx with the finger
or a blunt object. Ipecac syrup can be given in a dose of 10
to 15 ml and can be repeated in 15 to 30 minutes if
emesis does not occur. Water should be given after
administration of ipecac syrup.

The victim of an inhaled poison should be removed
immediately from the gas, vapor, aerosol, or dust. Adequate ventilation must be ensured.

Carbon Monoxide Poisoning

The organs that are most sensitive to carbon monoxide poisoning and the resultant arterial oxygen deficit
are the brain and heart. The patient may present with
various neurological deficits, seizures, or coma. Cerebral
edema may develop as well. Arrhythmias and myocardial infarction may occur. The patient may have pink or
cherry colored skin and mucous membranes.

Treatment for carbon monoxide poisoning includes
removal from the toxic environment and ventilation
with 100% oxygen. If a hyperbaric chamber is available,
this mode of treatment should be considered, even several hours after the inhalation of carbon monoxide.

Salicylate Poisoning

Salicylates can directly stimulate the respiratory
center, with resultant hyperventilation and respiratory
alkalosis. If toxic levels of salicylates persist, metabolic
acidosis develops. At this point the patient is usually in a
coma.

If the patient is awake, attempt to determine what
drugs he has taken. Have other persons present look for
and collect any containers that might have held medications.

When several drugs have been ingested they often
have antagonistic actions; therefore, the pupillary size
and reactivity are often useless indicators of the patient's
physical status.

Management of salicylate intoxication consists of
gastric lavage, since salicylates can remain in the gas-

trointestinal tract for prolonged periods. Dehydration must be corrected by intravenous administration of lactated Ringer's solution, 500 ml per hour. Maintenance of an adequate airway is important.

Barbiturate Poisoning

Barbiturates, other sedatives, and alcohol, which are often used concurrently, depress the central nervous system. A patent airway and adequate oxygenation must be maintained as well as support of circulation. Gastric lavage should be performed.

Psychotropic Drug Overdosage

With the increasing use of drugs having atropine-like activity, more patients are seen with atropine psychoses and comas. These drugs include antidepressants, antihistamines, antiparkinsonians, and some antipsychotics. Signs and symptoms of atropine toxicity and coma are delirium, tachycardia, absence of bowel sounds, warm dry skin, hyperthermia, and decrease in secretions. Cardiac arrhythmias occur with massive overdoses.

Physostigmine is a specific antidote for this type of poisoning. The dosage is 1 to 2 mg intramuscularly every 30 minutes to 3 hours. Slowing of heart rate and an increase in bowel sounds are the most sensitive indicators of physostigmine action.

Narcotic Overdose

When there is possible drug overdose and respirations are depressed, naloxone (Narcan) can be given to quickly determine if the offending drug is a narcotic. The usual dose is 0.4 mg intravenously, repeated every three or four minutes until the respiratory rate is greater than eight breaths per minute. If no response is noted after two or three doses, look for other causes of the respiratory depression.

Drug-Induced Parkinsonism

People who have been placed on antipsychotic medication may develop sudden side effects. These include parkinsonian movements, dystonias, torticollis, and oculogyric crises. These people need reassurance that the symptoms are distressing but not life threatening. Intramuscular or intravenous benztropine (Cogentin) or diphenhydramine (Benadryl) will relieve the symptoms within 5 to 30 minutes. The usual route for treating acute dystonia is intramuscular or intravenous, followed by oral maintenance doses. The usual dosage of benztropine is 2 mg intramuscularly or intravenously, then 2 mg three times a day by mouth; the usual dosage of diphenhydramine is 50 mg intramuscularly or intravenously followed by 50 mg two or three times a day orally.

HYPERTENSIVE CRISIS

Hypertensive crisis is an uncommon state of sudden elevation of the diastolic blood pressure to levels usually greater than 120 mm Hg. Renal failure is invariably present to some degree, and symptoms include headache, convulsions, transient focal neurological deficits, nausea, vomiting, stupor, and often coma.

Hypertensive crisis is an acute medical emergency requiring immediate treatment. The treatment of choice is intravenous diazoxide (Hyperstat), which has an immediate onset of action following a rapid intravenous injection of 300 mg in adults. Blood pressure will usually return toward pretreatment level within two to six hours.

ALTERED CONSCIOUSNESS

When a patient appears to be in an altered state of consciousness, an assessment of his vital signs will indicate the urgency of the situation and can also serve as a baseline to determine improvement or deterioration. The examiner should note the color of the skin, the odor of the breath, and the size and reactivity of the pupils and should carefully examine the patient for evidence of injury. The AVPU system is easy to remember and is a quick guide to consciousness assessment. The patient is judged to be Alert; responsive to Verbal stimuli; responsive to Painful stimuli; or Unresponsive.

Coma and stupor are two different states of unconsciousness. In coma the patient cannot be aroused and will exhibit only a reflex response to painful stimuli. In stupor a patient who is vigorously stimulated will react with behavior that indicates some awareness of his surroundings.

Behavioral Problems in Old Age

There are two types of changes in mentation in the elderly. In *senile brain disease,* there is a gradual deterioration of the mental faculties over an extended period of time, and the person is not aware of the loss. These people usually attract attention by getting lost and by believing that they or others are someone else. In *cerebral arteriosclerosis*, the blood vessels are affected and there is a deficient supply of nutrients to the brain. This condition is more abrupt in onset and tends to fluctuate over time. The person is usually acutely aware that he is losing his mental faculties. He may try to hide the defect from others, becoming more anxious, depressed, and possibly suicidal.

Alcohol Intoxication

Alcohol is a common cause of altered mental states, but the odor of alcohol does not prove that it is the cause of coma nor does it exclude other etiologies. Trauma is not uncommon in alcoholism. The patient may also have taken barbiturates or other sedatives. Supportive treatment is indicated when acute ethanol intoxication presents without complications. If there is a previous history of chronic alcoholism, the patient may develop seizures or hallucinations (delirium tremens). During transport to the hospital the patient must be gently restrained and should be turned on his side to prevent aspiration in case he vomits.

Diabetic Ketoacidosis

Ketoacidosis can be an early or late manifestation of diabetes. It may be precipitated by acute infection, omission of insulin or oral hypoglycemic agents, acute emotional upset, or long-standing poorly controlled diabetes. The patient may present early with excess thirst and urination, anorexia, and, perhaps, nausea and vomiting. Later he may develop hyperventilation and abdominal pain, and physical examination will reveal signs of dehydration. The breath may have an acetone odor.

Hypotonic saline should be infused at a rate of 1000 ml per hour with 50 units of regular insulin. A careful log of the state of consciousness, fluid intake, and urine output should be maintained. With the administration of insulin and correction of the acidosis, potassium will shift out of the serum and hypokalemia may develop, manifest by hyporeflexia, paresthesias, and respiratory depression. Potassium supplements should be started only after an adequate urine output is present.

Hyperosmolar nonketotic coma is an unusual disturbance of glucose metabolism, in which the patient may present in stupor or coma. It most often occurs in elderly patients with mild, adult onset diabetes. There is no acetone odor on the breath. Treatment consists of the administration of normal saline, 500 ml per hour, in addition to small doses (10 units) of insulin. Patients are often exquisitely sensitive to insulin in this state.

Hypoglycemia

In hypoglycemia, blood glucose is less than 50 mg/100 ml because the glucose is being abnormally utilized. The patient may have hunger, nausea, lethargy, frequent yawning, or even seizures or coma. Whenever hypoglycemia is suspected a blood sample should be drawn for glucose determination, and 50 ml of 50% glucose should be administered intravenously.

Renal Failure

A patient with renal insufficiency may be only mildly confused or may present in a coma. On examination the patient may appear physically normal or may look pale and sallow and have "uremic frost," a white deposit on and around the lips.

Renal failure has prerenal, renal, and postrenal causes, and each of these can be either acute or chronic. Decreasing circulating blood volume or hypotension causes acute *prerenal failure*, which can be diagnosed by signs of hypovolemia.

Renal failure can be acute such as an acute tubular necrosis, which may be related to ischemia or nephrotoxins. It can also be cortical in origin, which as a rule is not caused by hypotension or hypovolemia but by vascular problems such as a dissecting aneurysm.

Postrenal failure is usually caused by obstruction of the urinary tract.

Treatment of renal failure depends on its etiology (prerenal, renal, or postrenal) and nature (acute or chronic). Careful examination of the blood pressure with the patient in recumbent and standing positions or, if not feasible, sitting will help to test for hypovolemia. Placement of a catheter in the urinary bladder will assist in the evaluation of a prostatic source of obstruction.

If the patient is felt to be hypovolemic with resultant prerenal failure, a fluid challenge should be given in the hospital in conjunction with a diuretic, if necessary. Careful attention to fluid and electrolyte balance is of the utmost importance. If the patient develops a "diuretic phase" it will be necessary to increase sodium and water intake. Urinary catheters should be removed as soon as possible, since they are a focus of infection.

If the renal failure is felt to be chronic in origin, a fluid challenge should not be given unless there is strong evidence that the patient is indeed hypovolemic.

Hepatic Failure

Coma resulting from hepatic failure is not difficult to diagnose in the chronically jaundiced patient with an obviously distended abdomen due to ascites. These specific findings may not be present in patients who have recently developed hepatic insufficiency with resultant coma. The patient may have scleral icterus, small vascular eruptions (spider nevi) that blanch with pressure, and enlargement of the liver or spleen. If the hands are held in extension there may be a peculiar flap. Other causes of coma should be excluded, particularly acute alcohol intoxication or trauma.

Supportive fluid therapy is started while the patient is being transported to the emergency department. **Gastrointestinal bleeding**, which is an emergency, is a frequent accompaniment.

p. 63

Respiratory Failure

Patients with pulmonary insufficiency may develop changes in mentation or even coma. The evaluation and treatment of respiratory emergencies are outlined in Chapter 3.

Acute Adrenal Insufficiency

Sudden cessation of long-term steroid therapy results in hypotension, nausea, vomiting, abdominal pain, hypovolemia, or a change in mental status. It is important to determine the patient's usual steroid dose before treatment, which consists of correction of the hypovolemia with 1000 ml per hour of lactated Ringer's solution and administration of 100 mg of hydrocortisone intravenously. Further treatment should be directed by a physician.

Hyperthyroid Crisis

Various types of neurological abnormalities, including psychoses, convulsions, or coma, may be seen in hyperthyroid crisis or so-called "thyroid storm." The patient usually appears agitated, the skin is warm and flushed, and the pulse is fast and may be irregular. There may be an enlarged thyroid gland; exophthalmos may be present. Treatment consists of infusing lactated Ringer's solution, 1000 ml per hour, during transport.

Myxedema Coma

Myxedema is the most severe form of hypothyroidism, in which the patient becomes lethargic, and may progress to a stuporous condition known as myxedema coma. The usual signs of thyroid hormone deficiency (puffiness of the eyes, face, and extremities) will be present in these patients. Myxedema coma is usually not an emergency, but patients may be hypothermic and should be covered with blankets during transport to the hospital. These patients are prone to congestive heart failure because of a large flabby heart and should be transported with the head of the stretcher elevated.

Electrolyte Imbalance

Electrolyte imbalance, especially hyponatremia, should be considered in patients with altered mentation. *Hyponatremia* is most commonly dilutional in origin and is seen in patients with excessive total body water such as in edema, ascites, or congestive heart failure. Restriction of water intake is the most important initial management measure. Hyponatremia can be caused by the combination of a low-sodium diet and diuretic therapy.

Hypernatremia almost always results from a loss of water, most often in patients who are stuporous or have some other disability that prevents them from responding normally to thirst. Treatment consists of water, either orally or in the form of 5% glucose intravenously.

CENTRAL NERVOUS SYSTEM INFECTION

Patients presenting with headache, neck ache, vomiting, and photophobia should be suspected of having a central nervous system infection. The temperature is commonly elevated and there is usually resistance to flexion of the neck on examination. This flexion resistance is differentiated from cervical muscle spasm by the fact that the head can be moved from side to side quite easily in most cases of infection. With meningitis, the hips and knees may flex in response to attempts to flex the neck (Brudzinski's sign). An infusion of lactated Ringer's solution will help overcome dehydration during transport to the hospital.

CEREBROVASCULAR DISEASE

The diagnosis of a *cerebrovascular accident* (stroke) should be suspected in the presence of complete or partial paralysis (especially one-sided) with aphasia. There may be loss of consciousness, and other vital signs may or may not be altered.

Subarachnoid hemorrhage usually causes sudden severe headache and neck pain, rapidly followed by coma. Treatment of patients with either type of cerebrovascular disease consists of lactated Ringer's solution and rapid transport to the hospital.

INTERMITTENT CEREBROVASCULAR INSUFFICIENCY

Patients who complain of light-headedness and momentary instability when they arise from a recumbent or sitting position and who have other transient difficulties, such as momentary aphasia, amnesia, and ataxia, are likely to be experiencing intermittent cerebrovascular insufficiency. No emergency treatment is necessary.

BITES AND STINGS

Bee, Wasp, and Ant Stings

The most common stings are those of the bee and wasp. The bee leaves its stinger in the skin, and the wasp (or hornet) injects the poison and withdraws the stinger. The local reaction to the sting usually consists of pain, swelling, and itching or burning. In the event of **anaphylactic reaction**, death can occur within minutes.

p. 105

Ant bites most often occur when a person sits or stands where ants are numerous. The usual local reaction is pain with swelling. An anaphylactic reaction can occur but is rare.

Local treatment of insect stings consists of the application of cold packs and, in the case of bee stings, careful scraping of the site to remove the stinger. Grasping the stinger with forceps in an effort to remove it may cause further injection of venom.

Scorpion Stings

Most scorpion stings are minor and will not produce a serious reaction. There may be local pain and swelling, which is treated by applying cold packs or washing the area with ammonia. One species of scorpion found in Arizona may produce an anaphylactic reaction, which can result in death. Treatment consists of local cold application, maintenance of an airway, and support of respiration as needed. An antivenom is available against the poison of this species.

Spider Bites

Whenever possible, the type of spider should be identified. Care must be taken to prevent further bites during this effort. The majority of spider bites are only locally irritating, but those of the black widow and the brown recluse can be more serious.

Persons bitten by the black widow spider may not be aware of the bite until symptoms begin to show an hour or so later. The bite produces two small skin punctures. Systemic symptoms include muscle cramps in the back spreading to the abdomen, tightness of the chest, and difficulty breathing. There may be nausea and vomiting. Treatment consists of maintaining an airway, supporting respiration, and administering antivenom. Death from this type of bite is rare.

The brown recluse spider is usually found in wood piles and sheds where there is little activity. The bite may not be recognized immediately, and local redness and swelling are seen after a few hours. Later manifestations are local slough and a draining ulcer. Death from the bite is rare.

Snake Bites

Identification of the snake is helpful, but there may be danger in trying to capture it. Any snake with rattles is poisonous. The coral snake has red, yellow, and black rings and may be distinguished from similar snakes by the relationship of the rings. The red and yellow rings are next to each other on a coral snake. If the red rings are next to the black rings, the snake is not poisonous.

The bite of the coral snake does not produce fang marks; the snake chews instead of bites, and the venom is on the surface of the wound. The area should be flooded with water, and incisions should not be made.

If there is direct intravascular injection of venom at the time of the bite, venom spreads throughout the body in a short time and can cause death in spite of treatment.

Local findings in addition to the fang marks will often be severe pain and swelling. Systemic findings will normally be seen within the first two hours. If none are seen by that time, the likelihood of their occurrence is not great. The systemic symptoms consist of nausea, vomiting, weakness, sweating, tachycardia, and hypertension. The use of antivenom is indicated in persons who develop these systemic symptoms. There is a significant incidence of side effects from antivenom, which furthermore is not of value as a local injection. Allergic reactions are common, and fatal anaphylaxis has occurred. Steroids are best reserved for those patients in whom significant reactions to the antivenom are seen.

Immediate Treatment

The best management immediately following a snake bite is application of a cold compress over the bite and placement of a snug tourniquet between the bite and the heart. The tourniquet should not be loosened unless swelling progresses above it. The tourniquet should only be tight enough to prevent the spread of venom and not so tight as to shut off arterial circulation.

Later Treatment

Whether a tourniquet has been applied or not, a longitudinal incision should be made through the fang marks and the *skin only*. Suction should then be applied. The use of a suction device such as a rubber cup or a cut-off syringe is best. The mouth can be used if there are no open sores, but this greatly increases the danger of infection. Direct local excision of the bite area with primary closure is sometimes indicated; immediate transport to a hospital is necessary in these situations.

Human Bites

What appears to be a minor wound on the hand from a fight can become severely infected. No matter how insignificant, such a wound must be regarded as potentially dangerous. Surgical consultation must be obtained.

Animal Bites

Management of animal bites is the same as that of human bites — surgical advice. A primary concern in the case of bites by dogs and many wild animals is that the animal may have rabies. Many dogs have been inoculated, but those that have not must be observed, after being caged or tied, for 10 to 14 days after biting someone. Should the dog have rabies and be infective, it will die within this period.

Signs of rabies infection in humans are paresthesia, tingling or pain in the area of the bite or in the affected extremity, headache, stiff neck, malaise, lethargy, and seizures. After the patient begins to show signs of rabies, treatment is generally ineffective and death follows despite intense supportive care.

Marine Animal Bites and Stings

Table 10–1 MARINE ANIMAL INJURIES AND TREATMENT

Animal	Habitat	Symptoms	Treatment
Stingray	Tropical waters of most seas; some warmer temperate waters near Southern California and Gulf of Mexico; river systems of South America, Africa, and Southeastern Asia.	Intense spreading local pain; syncope, nausea, weakness, anxiety common; vomiting, diarrhea, sweating, fasciculations, cramps, respiratory distress in some instances.	Cleanse thoroughly; remove any part of barb remaining in wound; soak affected area in hot water 30–60 minutes; meat tenderizer may help destroy toxin; analgesics such as meperidine for pain; suture wound if necessary; tetanus prophylaxis advised.
Scorpion fish	Temperate and tropic zones of all seas; the most venomous, the stonefish, occurring in the tropical Indo-Pacific.	Immediate, intense, rapidly spreading pain, same as with stingray; conjunctivitis; cyanosis; swelling of regional lymph nodes.	Hot water and local care as for stingray.
Jellyfish Portuguese man-of-war Sea anemones Corals	Atlantic Coast and Indo-Pacific region.	Pain as stinging or burning sensation; muscular cramps, dyspnea, nausea, vomiting, weakness, anaphylaxis; some fatalities (Australia).	Apply aromatic spirits of ammonia or alcohol in a compress to deactivate or "fix" the nematocyst and prevent further stinging; meat tenderizer also reported to deactivate toxin; after 15 minutes, scrape off inactivated tentacles (application of powder aids

			scraping); 10 ml of 10 per cent calcium gluconate IV will help relieve muscular cramps, or use muscle relaxants. Coral cuts heal slowly with frequent infections; clean wound and apply antibiotic ointment.
Sea urchin	Warm waters around pilings, rocks, wrecks.	Local pain, redness, swelling, intense burning, occasional dizziness; transient muscular palsies.	Remove spines with forceps; look for embedded tips, which must be excised surgically if not absorbed within 48 hours; purple discoloration from spines at site of injury not dangerous; warm water relieves symptoms.
Squid Octopus	Temperate and tropical waters.	Local pain, swelling, burning, redness, free bleeding from wound.	General supportive care.
Barracuda Sharks	Florida, West Indies, Brazil, Indo-Pacific region. Shores and open waters.	Blood loss from lacerations or bites, as indicated.	Shock prevention; tourniquet to control bleeding; prompt suture of wounds; tetanus prophylaxis and antibiotics.
Moray eel	Tropical seas and near reefs.	Blood loss from wound.	Wound irrigation; hemostasis; wound suture; tetanus prophylaxis and antibiotics.
Electric fish Rays	Tropics in fresh water. Temperate and tropic ocean.		No treatment required, except to control panic and possibly assist swimmer to shore.

RADIATION INJURY

Exposure to radioactive material most commonly occurs in accidents involving the hauling of such material or in plants where it is used. Radioactivity cannot be seen or felt, and personnel may be exposed to relatively high levels of radiation for considerable lengths of time without being aware of the danger. Think of the radiation injury possible when accidents involve vehicles carrying radioactive material, even if the victims appear uninjured.

Prevention of further contamination is paramount. Spectators should be kept out of the area, and victims should be promptly removed. Radioactive contamination can be picked up on the clothing, shoes, and exposed skin of victims and rescue personnel. Clothing worn while in the accident area should be removed as soon as possible and kept isolated until it can be properly decontaminated. The patient should be taken to the emergency department and thoroughly washed to remove all radioactive material.

NEAR DROWNING

p. 43   Any person who appears to have drowned should receive **cardiopulmonary resuscitation**. Mouth-to-mouth resuscitation efforts can be started while the patient is still in the water. External cardiac compression should follow as soon as the patient can be placed on a firm surface. Keeping the patient warm is equally important but should not preclude the immediate initiation of CPR. Once spontaneous respiration is established, the patient is transported to the emergency department for evaluation.

HYPOTHERMIA

Loss of body heat caused by exposure to extreme cold will result in uncontrolled shivering, confusion, and cardiac arrhythmias. The patient will ultimately die without treatment. Inadequate or wet clothing and high wind velocities increase the loss of body heat.

The field treatment of hypothermia includes removing the wet clothes and placing the patient in a dry environment. In the hospital, if the core temperature is greater than 32° C, peripheral warming utilizes warm humidified oxygen (40° C), warm intravenous fluids, and, possibly, warmed nasogastric irrigation. Close monitoring for arrhythmias and respiratory difficulties is mandatory. When the core temperature is below 32° C internal rewarming is accomplished by either peritoneal dialysis with warm saline dialysate or, if cardiac arrest has occurred, cardiopulmonary bypass. Rewarming may take 12 to 24 hours.

During external rewarming there is an increased risk of ventricular fibrillation and so-called "rewarming shock." This is caused by an increased lactic acid and potassium load from the tissues in which anaerobic metabolism had been taking place during the hypothermia.

DECOMPRESSION SICKNESS

Decompression sickness is caused by a rapid drop of air pressure, as in flying at high altitudes or ascending from a deep underwater dive. Symptoms may consist of pain in the joints, ears, and bowel, loss of vision, dizziness, paralysis, convulsions or unconsciousness, choking, and shortness of breath. The symptoms may have their onset immediately or as much as five or six hours later.

Repressurization should be accomplished as rapidly as possible. Anyone who is responsible for such a patient should know the location of the closest repressurization tank and have rate-of-ascent tables available. A central registry of repressurization tanks is available by dialing "512-LEOFAST."

obstetrical emergencies

Medical emergencies in pregnant women require special consideration. First, there are two patients involved, mother and fetus. Second, the fetus is at great risk in any situation that results in poor utero-placental perfusion such as hypovolemia, supine hypotension (compression of the aorta and vena cava by the uterus), cardiac failure, or hypoxemia, including a decrease in ambient oxygen from an unpressurized aircraft, carbon monoxide poisoning, or mountain climbing at high altitudes.

During pregnancy, there is an increase in cardiac output, blood volume, heart rate, renal blood flow, and glomerular filtration. These increases begin in the first trimester and reach levels of 30 to 40 per cent above nonpregnant values by the latter part of the second trimester.

There is a generalized smooth muscle relaxation in pregnancy, producing peripheral vascular dilation, poor gastrointestinal tract muscle tone (constipation), increased blood flow through all organs (headaches, sinus congestion, epistaxis, hemoptysis, bladder irritability, and urinary frequency), and relaxation of the diaphragm (dyspepsia and heartburn).

Persons attending women of childbearing age in emergency situations should always keep in mind that the patient might be pregnant. If the patient is alert she should always be asked about the possibility of pregnancy. Many patients, particularly in the early weeks of pregnancy, may not be aware of the condition or may not think it important to volunteer this information. If the last menstrual period was more than 30 days ago or if the period was abnormal in any way, pregnancy complications should be included in the differential diagnosis.

The normal duration of pregnancy is 40 weeks, counting from the first day of the last menstrual period. If the patient's uterus is at or below the umbilicus, if she has not felt fetal movement, or if the uterus is not palpable but she strongly suspects she is pregnant, the pregnancy is of less than 20 weeks' duration. If the patient's uterus is palpable above the umbilicus and she has been aware of fetal movement, the pregnancy has proceeded beyond the twentieth week.

COMPLICATIONS OF THE FIRST HALF OF PREGNANCY

Hyperemesis Gravidarum (Intractable Vomiting)

Persistent nausea and vomiting with resultant dehydration and ketosis may complicate early pregnancy. One of the distinguishing features of hyperemesis of pregnancy is that the patient usually complains of being quite hungry. Other conditions that must be considered when hyperemesis is present are acute viral gastrointestinal infection, hepatitis, bowel obstruction, acute cholecystitis, and acute pancreatitis.

A patient with intractable vomiting should be hospitalized to exclude the other diagnostic possibilities and to rapidly hydrate the patient and reestablish normal electrolyte balance. An intravenous infusion of lactated Ringer's solution should be started.

Abdominal or Pelvic Pain with Vaginal Bleeding

The most common cause of abdominal and pelvic pain in the first 20 weeks of pregnancy is spontaneous abortion. If midline lower abdominal cramping pain is noted, especially radiating into the back, and if there is significant vaginal bleeding (equal to or greater than that of the patient's menstrual period), spontaneous abortion is very likely the source.

If the patient complains of lateral lower abdominal or pelvic pain and if the pain radiates into the flank or into the lower extremities, adnexal disease, such as hemorrhage into or torsion of an ovarian cyst, or ectopic (tubal) pregnancy must be suspected. These conditions are usually associated with less vaginal bleeding than that found in spontaneous abortion. Other causes of vaginal hemorrhage are carcinoma of the cervix, lacerations of the vagina or cervix, and severe infections of the cervix.

The correct diagnosis is the key in the treatment of patients with acute abdominal or pelvic pain and vaginal bleeding. If the patient's pain is midline and cramping, the bleeding is minimal, and the vital signs are stable, she can be transported to a hospital with an intravenous infusion. However, if ectopic pregnancy or a ruptured corpus luteum cyst is suspected, significant hemorrhage can occur. These patients should be transported without delay, preferably with an intravenous infusion of lactated Ringer's solution, 500 ml per hour. An anti-shock garment is useful in controlling hemorrhage during transport. If pain requires an analgesic, 25 to 50 mg of meperidine (Demerol) should be given intravenously. Blood clots expressed from the vagina should be examined, and any tissue present should be sent to the pathologist for examination.

Syncope

The most frequent cause of syncope in the first half of pregnancy is hyperventilation. The patient first notices tingling about the mouth, numbness of the hands, and a sensation of breathlessness occasionally accompanied by nausea. These symptoms frequently begin in crowded places.

Patients recovering from a syncopal episode and whose vital signs are within normal limits usually need only reassurance. If episodes are recurrent or if vital signs are abnormal, including an increase in pulse rate and a decrease in blood pressure, or if the pulse is irregular, the patient should be hospitalized to rule out cardiac disease and to detect hypoglycemia. Hospitalization also allows observation of the patient before, during, and immediately after a syncopal episode to detect any characteristic signs of neurological disease.

Instructing the patient to rebreath carbon dioxide by placing a small paper bag over the nose and mouth will often provide prompt relief from recurrent episodes of hyperventilation.

COMPLICATIONS OF THE SECOND HALF OF PREGNANCY

Efforts should be made to avoid hypoxia of the fetus at any gestational age, but at about 26 to 28 weeks' gestation extrauterine survival of the fetus becomes a viable possibility. In any emergency involving a woman in the latter half of pregnancy (during which time premature labor and delivery is a possibility), consideration should be given to transporting the patient to a hospital that provides a full range of perinatal intensive care. The following general measures are vital in the emergency treatment of a woman in the latter half of pregnancy:

1. Maintain an adequate airway and increase ambient oxygen to ensure maximum oxygen transport across the placenta. There is no danger to the normal fetus in increasing maternal arterial oxygen.

2. Whenever possible, keep the mother in the lateral recumbent position to avoid supine hypotension. If she must be on her back, elevate the right hip with a rolled sheet or blanket.

3. Maintain adequate circulating blood volume by an infusion of lactated Ringer's solution, 500 ml per hour.

4. If transport in an unpressurized aircraft over 8000 ft is absolutely necessary, administer oxygen.

5. Monitor fetal heart rate with a battery-operated ultrasound detector. A fetal heart rate of 120 to 160 beats per minute is normal. Fetal bradycardia or tachycardia must be considered a sign of fetal distress.

Hemorrhage

Vaginal bleeding described by the patient as equal to or greater than a menstrual flow must always be regarded as ominous in the second half of pregnancy. This bleeding must be distinguished from "bloody show," which is the bloody mucous discharge frequently noted in the latter weeks of pregnancy. Vaginal and cervical lesions can cause bleeding in the second trimester, but the bleeding is usually utero-placental in origin. About one-third of the cases of significant late pregnancy bleeding are due to placenta previa, a condition in which all or a portion of the cervix is covered by a low-lying placenta. This bleeding is usually painless and can often be profuse.

Another third of the cases of significant late pregnancy bleeding are due to premature separation of a normally implanted placenta (abruptio placentae). This condition, which is associated with very high fetal and neonatal death rates, can be distinguished by pain, uterine contractions, and uterine tenderness commonly accompanying the bleeding. The remaining third of the cases are due to hemorrhage from the margin of the placenta, or, very rarely, from an abnormal feto-placental blood vessel extending over the cervix (vasa previa).

Blood samples should be drawn for a complete blood count, coagulation studies, and cross-match, and an intravenous infusion of lactated Ringer's solution should be started with a 16-gauge needle. Fetal heart rate as well as maternal blood pressure and pulse should be monitored frequently. The mother should be maintained in the lateral recumbent position, and oxygen should be administered.

Under no circumstances should manual examination

of the vagina be done in cases of late pregnancy hemor-rhage. This can cause disruption of a low-lying placenta with resultant catastrophic hemorrhage. A manual examination should only be performed in an operating room where all the facilities for blood transfusion and immediate cesarean section are available.

Rupture of Membranes and Premature Labor

About one pregnant woman in ten will experience rupture of fetal membranes prior to the onset of labor. Premature rupture of membranes does not always imply a premature birth. The dangers of this complication are prolapse of the umbilical cord and infection resulting in amnionitis and possible fetal sepsis and pneumonia. A painless vaginal discharge of watery fluid is the usual symptom of premature rupture.

Other conditions that may masquerade as leakage of amniotic fluid are urinary stress incontinence, which is not uncommon in the last half of pregnancy, and vaginitis or cervicitis with profuse loss of fluid from the vagina.

All patients in the second half of pregnancy who complain of water fluid loss from the vagina must be considered to have ruptured fetal membranes until the diagnosis can be confirmed or excluded by vaginal examination with a sterile speculum. Detection of a fetal heart rate of between 120 and 160 beats per minute without decelerations below 100 beats per minute excludes significant cord occlusion. No additional examination is necessary until the patient can be evaluated with a speculum to confirm the diagnosis.

The latent period between the rupture of membranes and the onset of labor is greater than 24 hours in most patients who have not reached 36 weeks' gestation. This time is valuable in arranging transport of the mother to an adequate perinatal facility. If labor has not begun, the patient may travel in an automobile without special attendants. If labor has begun or if there is any evidence of amnionitis (fever, maternal pulse over 100, fetal heart rate over 160, or uterine tenderness), the mother should be transported by the most expedient conveyance with constant attendance by trained personnel.

In cases in which uterine contractions have begun, drugs to inhibit labor may be considered by the physician who will eventually care for the patient. Intravenous alcohol is sometimes administered in emergency transport situations. A 10% solution of ethyl alcohol in 5% dextrose is administered at a rate of 15 ml/kg of maternal body weight over a two-hour period (loading dose), followed by a maintenance infusion rate of 1.5 mg/kg/hr. The patient will usually become sedated and somnolent; on occasion she will be agitated or even combative. Urinary incontinence is occasionally a problem, and hypotension, nausea, and vomiting may occur. The patient should be given 30 ml of an antacid prior to the alcohol infusion and placed in the left or right lateral decubitus position to maximize uterine blood flow and to avoid aspiration in the event of vomiting. If the patient becomes obtunded, the alcohol infusion should be discontinued. Other labor-inhibiting drugs should be given only after consultation with a physician.

Seizures

Preeclampsia, a disease of unknown etiology occurring in pregnant women, produces generalized vasospasm and results in hypertension, proteinuria, edema, and, in its most severe form, cerebral edema, convulsions (at which time it is called eclampsia), fetal death, and, occasionally, maternal death. Seizures of eclampsia rarely occur in the absence of other signs of preeclampsia. Other diagnostic possibilities are idiopathic epilepsy, central nervous system thrombosis or hemorrhage, hypoglycemia, and drug overdose.

As with any other seizure patient, the pregnant woman who has a seizure must be evaluated immediately to ensure a patent airway and adequate ventilation and circulation. If any of these processes are compromised, standard measures to correct them must be instituted without delay, including tilting the head, supporting the chin, suctioning secretions or vomitus, inserting an oral airway, endotracheal intubation, oxygen administration, infusion of intravenous fluids, or even cardiopulmonary resuscitation when required. If repeated seizures occur, diazepam (Valium)is the drug of choice, 5 mg intravenously. All seizure patients should have blood samples drawn for electrolyte and blood sugar determinations or drug assays, their vital signs monitored frequently, and an intravenous infusion of lactated Ringer's solution begun. They should be transported at once to a hospital.

If hypertension is detected and the patient is suspected of having eclampsia, 4 gm of magnesium sulfate in a 20% solution should be given intravenously slowly over a 10-minute period. If transport to a hospital will take more than one hour, the magnesium sulfate administration should be continued at the rate of 1 gm/hr. A Foley catheter should be inserted in the bladder to monitor urinary output until arrival. Deep tendon reflexes should be checked frequently. If reflexes are hyperactive or if ankle clonus is present, the hourly dose of magnesium sulfate can be increased to 2 gm or more; if reflexes are depressed, the dose should be reduced. Because the drug is excreted almost exclusively by the kidneys, it should be used cautiously in patients with reduced renal output.

Prolapse of the Umbilical Cord

Umbilical cord prolapse may occur before or during labor following rupture of membranes. Umbilical cord prolapse is more common in breech than in vertex presentations. If it is suspected, fetal heart tones should be auscultated as soon as possible; if the heart rate is over 100 beats per minute, the patient should be moved to a hospital or, if in the hospital, to the operating suite with the utmost dispatch. The umbilical cord should not be palpated or manipulated nor should a vaginal examination be performed, because stimulation of the cord can result in umbilical artery spasm and decreased fetoplacental circulation.

If fetal heart rate is less than 100 beats per minute, umbilical cord compression by the presenting part must be suspected, and the patient should be placed in a steep Trendelenburg's position (head down). If this does not result in improved fetal heart rate, the patient can be moved to the knee-chest position and the examiner's gloved hand inserted into the vagina to help elevate the presenting part. Pulsations of the cord can be determined by gentle palpation. This manual palpation should be performed while the patient is being transported to a hospital facility where preparations for abdominal delivery are being made.

If fetal heart tones cannot be detected and if the prolapsed cord is pulseless, the fetus must be considered dead, and further efforts to save it are not required.

Shock

Shock or cardiovascular collapse may occur in pregnant women as a result of a complication directly related to the pregnancy, such as hemorrhage from a placenta previa, or as a result of a disease or an accident coincident with the pregnancy.

Shock should be managed in the pregnant as well as in the nonpregnant patient with prompt support including maintenance of a patent airway, administration of supplemental oxygen, and intravenous replacement of fluid volume using lactated Ringer's solution.

Blood loss resulting in shock is usually apparent from either uterine hemorrhage or other obvious signs of bleeding. Occasionally the bleeding is hidden, such as with a concealed retroplacental hemorrhage (concealed abruptio placentae) or in the more rare conditions of rupture of the uterus, spleen, or liver. There are usually other signs and symptoms present to suggest the diagnosis of concealed bleeding, including abdominal pain, tenderness, absent bowel sounds, uterine irritability and tenderness, and, frequently, signs of fetal distress with a fetal heart rate of less than 100 beats per minute. Emergency treatment of the patient in shock, however, is the same regardless of its etiology (see Chapter 4).

EMERGENCY DELIVERY

Ideally, every baby should be born in a setting where personnel and facilities are available to perform fetal monitoring, emergency cesarean section, and neonatal resuscitation and stabilization. However, there are circumstances in which, because of unexpectedly rapid labor or geographical isolation, delivery occurs outside a hospital. Those attending women about to give birth should be prepared to assist them and to resuscitate and support the newborn.

Equipment

The following supplies should be kept in the ambulance for emergency deliveries:

A small sterile pack containing surgical gloves, bulb syringe, umbilical tape or cord clamps, Mayo scissors, container for the placenta, several towels, 4 × 4 gauze sponges, and a large vaginal pack;

An Ambu bag fitted with an infant mask and a pressure gauge;

A flashlight;

Several 3-ml disposable syringes with 22-gauge needles; and

Oxytocin: several 1-ml vials of 10 units each; methylergonovine maleate (Methergine): vials of 0.2 mg; and meperidine.

Technique

Most presentations are cephalic, but a few will be breech. Delivery will not be spontaneous with a transverse lie or shoulder presentation, both of which rarely occur. If the personnel present have not had specific instructions and experience in delivery, the mother should be allowed to deliver spontaneously, with no attempts made to rotate or manually extract the baby.

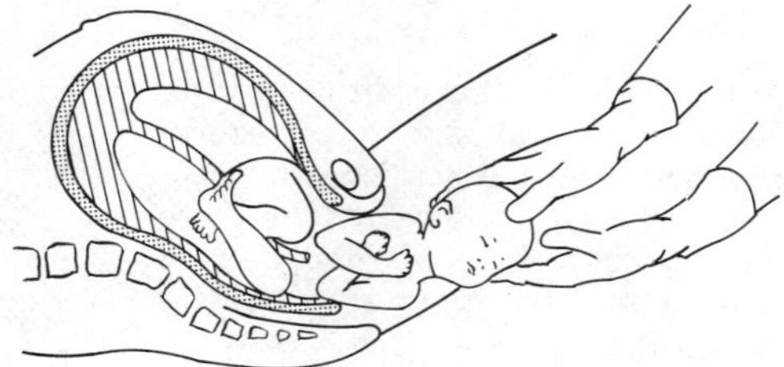

Figure 11–1 Supporting the baby's head during a spontaneous delivery.

Emergency personnel should support the baby's head during delivery (Fig. 11–1). Immediately after delivery, the infant's nares and oral pharynx should be gently aspirated with a bulb syringe to remove excess mucus. The infant is then dried gently with a sterile towel to minimize heat loss by evaporation. The umbilical cord is cut after being clamped or tied.

Resuscitation of the Infant

The first priority of care for the newborn is adequate respiration, manifested by breathing or crying. An infant with blue extremities in the first few minutes of life who is otherwise crying, breathing, and moving should not be regarded as abnormal. Adequate perfusion can be ascertained by a heart rate in excess of 100 beats per minute and a blue color beginning to turn pink, first in the trunk and head and last in the extremities. If the baby is pale, mottled, and has a heart rate under 100, circulation is inadequate; he should be immediately transported to a facility where cardiorespiratory resuscitation and blood transfusion are available.

Maintenance of the baby's body temperature is of the utmost importance to minimize oxygen consumption. This can be accomplished by wrapping the baby in a dry towel or blanket and holding it against the mother's body.

If respiration is not established in the first few

seconds after birth and there is poor muscle tone, no activity, and a heart rate below 100, the infant should be ventilated with the Ambu bag. The mask should be held gently but securely over the nose and mouth with the head in a military position (neck not hyperextended) and the chin supported with the fifth finger of the hand holding the mask on the face. Initial pressures required to inflate a neonate's lungs may be up to 80 ml of water. After several inflations of this magnitude, the baby should be ventilated with pressures of 20 ml of water at a rate of 20 breaths per minute. Adequate ventilation is evidenced by a pink central color, an increase in heart rate to over 100, and breath sounds heard bilaterally on auscultation. If an Ambu bag or an adequate substitute is not available, mouth-to-mouth ventilation can be used. The resuscitator's lips should cover both the nose and mouth of the infant, and the lungs should be inflated using only the pressure exerted by puffs from the cheeks.

Delivery of Placenta and Postpartum Hemorrhage

After the baby's condition has been deemed satisfactory, the mother should be reassessed. The placenta usually separates and delivers spontaneously into the vagina within 10 minutes after birth. In these cases, abdominal pressure by the mother or very gentle traction on the umbilical cord suffices to expel the placenta. No attempt should be made to deliver it by exaggerated, manual abdominal pressure or vigorous traction on the cord.

If the placenta is not expressed promptly or if there is profuse bleeding, an intravenous infusion of lactated Ringer's solution should be started and 30 units of oxytocin added to the infusion. The solution should be infused at a rate of 30 drops per minute or faster to maintain uterine tone and prevent excessive bleeding. If the placenta has not been expressed spontaneously within 30 minutes, manual removal is necessary in a hospital setting where blood transfusion, general anesthesia, and sterile instruments are available.

Once the placenta is expressed, uterine tone can be maintained by gentle massage over the fundus and the administration of oxytocin (30 units in 1000 ml of lactated Ringer's solution IV or 10 units [1 ml] IM). In nonhypertensive patients (BP not above 130/90), methyl-ergonovine maleate (Methergine), 0.2 mg intramuscularly, will help maintain uterine tone. Uterine atony is the most common cause of postpartum hemorrhage and is among the leading causes of maternal mortality.

If the placenta has delivered and the uterus is firm but vaginal hemorrhage persists, one must suspect a vaginal or cervical laceration. This can be detected and repaired only with adequate light, exposure, and surgical instruments; therefore, the patient must be transported promptly to a hospital. A sterile pack can be inserted into the vagina to tamponade the lacerated vessels. Meperedine may be required to relieve the pain of vaginal and perineal hematomas or the pressure of the vaginal pack until adequate surgical evaluation and repair can be performed.

POSTPARTUM COMPLICATIONS

Uterine Inversion

Inversion of the uterus can be recognized by a bulging red mass protruding from the vagina, with the placenta occasionally attached to its surface. This condition is frequently associated with extensive hemorrhage and shock. Immediate recognition of the condition, vigorous replacement of fluid volume, and prompt measures to reinvert the uterus are mandatory. An intravenous infusion of lactated Ringer's solution should be started immediately and transportation to a hospital initiated.

During transport, an effort can be made to encourage spontaneous reinversion. Using a gloved hand, the uterine fundus is gently but firmly pushed into the vagina and pressure is maintained over the fundus. In most cases a dimple will appear on the inverted fundus and reinversion will follow. The degree of hemorrhage and the consequent morbidity from uterine inversion are related directly to its duration.

Delayed Postpartum Hemorrhage

Following delivery, a period of involution of the uterus and healing of the placental site occurs, associated with the discharge of a small amount of blood and debris for up to five weeks. This vaginal discharge is ordinarily of about the same magnitude as a menstrual period. A few patients experience abnormally heavy bleeding; rarely, this is so profuse as to occasion a call for help or bring the patient to an emergency department. This bleeding occurs most commonly from 10 to 20 days after delivery. The placental eschar separates at this time, and the underlying endometrial vessels are not occluded by organizing thrombi. A short period of profuse, painless bleeding results. Frequently, by the time the patient has reached the office or emergency department, the dramatic bleeding has subsided.

Other causes of delayed abnormal postpartum bleeding are retained placental fragments, endometritis, and hemorrhage from a vaginal or cervical laceration or hematoma. The bleeding from retained placental fragments is more chronic and persistent, whereas the patient with endometritis will have lower abdominal pain and fever as well as a tender uterus. The possibility of vaginal or cervical lacerations or hematomas must be excluded by speculum and bimanual examinations.

Patients with delayed postpartum hemorrhage should have their vital signs monitored and a complete blood count performed. In most cases, treatment consists of methylergonovine maleate (Methergine), 0.2 mg every 4 hours by mouth for 24 hours. This stimulates uterine contractions, encouraging occlusion of any open vessels in the placental site until new thrombi can form. Occasionally, a blood transfusion will be necessary if the patient's signs and symptoms suggest hypovolemia. All patients should have speculum and bimanual pelvic evaluations to identify areas of cervical or vaginal trauma or infection. If the uterus is tender, endometritis must be suspected and the patient treated with antibiotics. If these measures do not control the excess bleeding, uterine curettage should be considered. Because of the danger of uterine scarring and endometrial adhesions (Asherman's syndrome) with curettage, this procedure is done only after more conservative approaches have failed.

special pediatric emergencies

Trauma is the main cause of death in children over the age of one year. Small children have limited ability to compensate for physiological derangement, and their clinical condition may deteriorate rapidly because of this. Therefore, emergency transportation techniques assume increased importance when a child is involved.

SPECIAL PHYSIOLOGICAL CONSIDERATIONS

Table 12–1 outlines normal vital signs and hourly urine output in various childhood age groups. Children who are anxious and upset usually have a somewhat elevated pulse rate and blood pressure.

Return of *skin color* to normal is a helpful guideline in adults and older children as a measure of the adequacy of peripheral circulation and cardiac output. Skin color may be a confusing sign in infants and small children, however, because they have a more labile peripheral circulation than adults. Small children are prone to peripheral vasoconstriction and mottling of the skin, especially if they are exposed and cold. When skin color returns to normal following resuscitation, it is a dependable sign that circulation has been adequately restored.

Table 12–1   NORMAL VITAL SIGNS BY AGE

Age	Respirations (breaths/min)	Heart (beats/min)	Blood Pressure	Urine Output (ml/hr)
First year	40	120	80/40	10
Years 1 to 5	30	100	110/60	20
Years 6 to 12	20	80	120/80	30

Special precautions must be taken in children to maintain body *temperature*. Children have a larger surface area compared with body weight than adults. They also have thinner skin and less subcutaneous fat, which results in an increased tendency to lose body heat. Hypothermia in infants can lead to severe acidosis and respiratory depression.

Children who are in pain or who are anxious usually hyperventilate; this often results in extreme *gastric dilatation*. Injured children may develop ileus as a result of decreased cardiac output. Diaphragmatic elevation caused by gastric or intestinal distention may interfere with respiration; the child already has a low pulmonary reserve as compared with an adult. Early passage of a nasogastric tube by the physician, nurse, or technician is an important consideration in any child with a severe injury or shock, especially if he is to be transported.

Blood volume in the infant and child is approximately 8 per cent of total body weight. Blood volume can be calculated by multiplying the measured or estimated weight in kilograms by 10 per cent. The latter figure is easier to remember than 8 per cent and works well, since hemorrhage is usually underestimated. A child in hypovolemic shock has lost at least one-fourth of his blood volume, which works out to be 10 ml per pound of body weight. A 1-unit transfusion in a child is approximately 5 ml per pound of body weight. These figures are helpful to those who treat both adults and children and who might otherwise be confused by size differences.

SPECIAL TECHNICAL CONSIDERATIONS

Airway

If the child is not breathing, tilt the head back and rapidly clear the pharynx of blood, secretions, or foreign bodies. Insert a pharyngeal airway and institute mouth-to-mouth breathing. Use a manually controlled artificial ventilation device as soon as possible. The mandible should be lifted forward so that the tongue, which is relatively large in a child, does not fall backward and obstruct the airway.

p. 19

Passing an **endotracheal tube** in a child requires proper size laryngoscope blades and endotracheal tubes in a variety of sizes. A simple guideline is to select a tube that will just fit in the child's nostril or one that approximates the breadth of the child's little fingernail (Fig. 12–1).

When passage of an endotracheal tube is not possible, tracheostomy must be considered. Although cricothyroidotomy is technically feasible in children, it may result in more long-standing laryngeal complications in this age group than in adults. The surgical approach to the trachea in the child is similar to that in an adult, except that certain precautions must be taken to avoid complications. The incision should be vertical, avoiding the first and second tracheal rings. No cross incisions need be made, and portions of cartilage should not be excised, since the trachea will then tend to collapse inward when the tube is removed and stricture may result.

Pneumothorax is an extremely common complication of emergency tracheostomy in children. Therefore, physical examination of the chest should be performed, and a chest x-ray should be obtained immediately following the procedure. It is always safest to perform a tracheostomy over an endotracheal tube or a pediatric bronchoscope.

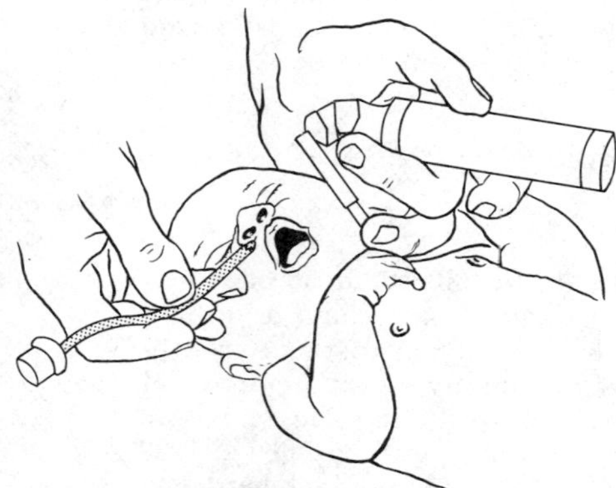

Figure 12–1 Selection of an endotracheal tube and use of a small laryngoscope.

If the heart is beating and the child is suffering primarily from hypovolemia, an intravenous cannula should be placed in any visible vein in an uninjured extremity. If an abdominal injury has occurred, it is preferable to select an intravenous route above the diaphragm. A plastic cannula may be placed either percutaneously or via a cutdown. Percutaneous subclavian catheters may be used in children, but one must take into account the fact that complications such as pneumothorax are more common in children under the age of six and in those who are restless and difficult to restrain.

If the patient is in shock due to bleeding, 10 ml per pound of body weight of lactated Ringer's solution should be administered rapidly over one hour while waiting for blood to be typed and cross-matched. If this infusion does not restore circulation, additional doses of 5 ml per pound of body weight per hour should be given. Children develop severe acidosis when in shock; therefore, 1 ml per pound of body weight of sodium bicarbonate solution should be given intravenously. Sodium bicarbonate ampules ordinarily contain 44 mEq per 50 ml, or about 1 mEq per ml.

If the heart is not beating, external cardiac compression should be started concurrent with ventilation. In cases of cardiac arrest, the child should be placed on his back on a firm surface, and external cardiac compression should be performed at a rate of 60 to 80 times per minute. Place the heel of the hand over the lower half of the sternum and compress the heart against the vertebral column in older children as in adults. The flat surface of two fingers is often sufficient pressure in small infants (Fig. 12–2).

The chest wall of infants and children is pliable, and the liver and spleen may be damaged if compression is too forceful. If peripheral pulses can be felt during external cardiac compression, the amount of force being applied is sufficient. If ventilation and external compression are adequate, a femoral pulse will be felt, peripheral circulation will improve, and dilated pupils will con-

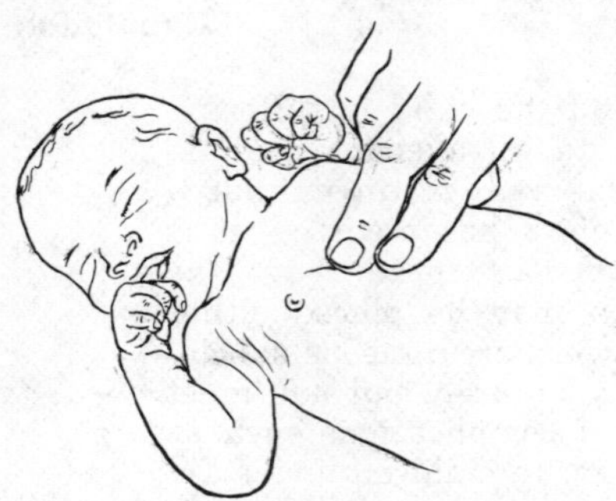

Figure 12–2 External cardiac compression in an infant.

strict. If these measures do not restore cardiac action and circulation, obtain an electrocardiogram and follow the usual resuscitative measures taken in adults (see Chapter 5).

CONDITIONS PECULIAR TO CHILDHOOD

Respiratory Disorders

In acute *asthmatic attacks,* the patient has difficulty exhaling and tends to have overexpansion of the chest. Aqueous epinephrine 1:1000 may be subcutaneously administered at a dose of 0.01 ml/kg of body weight. This may be repeated at 30-minute intervals for three doses as required. Methylprednisolone, 5 mg/kg of body weight, may also be given intravenously every four to six hours as required. Oxygen should be administered. Nebulized ethylnorepinephrine hydrochloride, 2 mg/ml (Bronkephrine) in a dose of 0.02 ml/kg of body weight, is also a helpful early measure. If the child is cyanotic, acidosis may be present; sodium bicarbonate, 1 ml/lb of body weight given intravenously, is then indicated. If respiratory obstruction continues, intubation or tracheostomy may be required.

Bronchiolitis is a viral infection of the lungs associated with both inspiratory and expiratory distress that ordinarily occurs in children younger than those who have asthma. Oxygen, intravenous methylprednisolone as indicated previously, and ethylnorepinephrine hydrochloride are helpful early measures.

Perhaps the most alarming respiratory difficulty in the childhood age group is *croup*, which is severe inspiratory obstruction of an emergent nature seen in children from age six months to four or five years. Humidified oxygen, intravenous methylprednisolone, and nebulized epinephrine may be helpful. Endotracheal intubation or even tracheostomy may occasionally be required. Although endotracheal intubation is preferable in cases of severe respiratory obstruction due to laryngotracheitis, the procedure is difficult to perform in children and should be done in the hospital by experienced personnel.

Children who have lesser degrees of respiratory obstruction and who are being managed expectantly from the standpoint of the airway must be kept from being overly active, since this may increase their respiratory distress. Small doses of a sedative may be appropriate, but extreme caution and moderation should be used in its administration.

Seizure Disorders

The child with decreased responsiveness and constant seizure activity is in danger of cardiorespiratory arrest and vomiting on aspiration. The patient should be protected from injury, and attention should be paid to the airway. Suction should be available to rid the nose and mouth of thick mucoid secretions ordinarily seen with increased salivation. Intravenous phenobarbital, 1 mg/kg of body weight, or diazepam (Valium), 2 mg intravenously in children over the age of one year, is helpful. Phenobarbital infusion may be repeated in 30 minutes to 1 hour if the first dose is insufficient. Phenytoin (Dilantin), 6 mg/kg intravenously, should be administered as well, although it will not act for several hours.

Ingestion of Poisons

Prior to initiating therapy, try to determine what the child has ingested. Respiratory obstruction or distress should be attended to first. Many communities have a poison control center, which can be reached by dialing "911" on the telephone.

If the ingestion has occurred shortly before the patient is seen, pass a nasogastric tube and lavage the stomach thoroughly with saline or water with the child on his right side to avoid aspiration if vomiting occurs. The ingestion of corrosives is an important exception to the recommendation of lavage, because lavage and vomiting might extend the damage. Children who have ingested corrosives may have airway problems from burns of the larynx. Clear the pharynx and mouth of poisonous particles.

In the case of ingestion of acid substances, instillation of about 100 ml of milk of magnesia or a dilute solution of sodium bicarbonate may be helpful after gastric lavage. Mild alkali ingestion may be treated with instillation of vinegar, but saline is probably easier to use.

An alternative method of preventing absorption of poisons is to induce vomiting. Syrup of ipecac, 15 ml in small children and 30 ml in children over 60 lb, is given by mouth, followed by large amounts of water. The patient is kept ambulatory, and if vomiting has not occurred in 15 minutes, the child may be stimulated to vomit with a suction catheter. Induced vomiting is contraindicated in the depressed patient who may have lost the gag reflex or in those who may have ingested strong acids, alkalis, or hydrocarbons such as kerosene.

If the patient is unresponsive and severely depressed, endotracheal intubation and assisted ventilation rather than stimulation are in order. Seizures may be treated as mentioned previously. Administration of antidotes is probably best deferred until the patient is hospitalized.

Child Abuse

The so-called battered child syndrome involves many forms of physical abuse and nutritional as well as psychological deprivation. These varying factors result in a clinical presentation which may be confusing and which may mimic other disease states. The characteristic finding is that the child has injuries of varying age, and it is invariably not possible to obtain a history sufficient to explain the injuries.

Most patients are under two years of age, and many will have signs of hygienic neglect in addition to injury. Multiple soft tissue injuries and burns are seen most commonly and ordinarily antedate the appearance of fractures or serious head injuries. Cigarette burns, multiple bruises, scars indicative of repetitive injury, and lacerations that cannot be explained on the basis of the history offered should arouse a suspicion of child abuse. Many children appear with serious head injuries or major internal injury and a history that is deliberately evasive. Application of the principles of airway maintenance and adequate resuscitation is the key to survival. When child abuse is suspected, it must be reported. The person reporting such abuse in good faith is protected by law in every state.

TRANSPORTATION OF THE NEONATE

Because of the tremendous expense involved in maintaining a neonatal intensive care center and the necessity of localizing experienced medical and associated personnel, newborns with emergency problems should be transported to special care centers. Many neonatal care centers now have mobile intensive care units. One of the essentials of emergency neonatal care is speed, but safety is clearly the major consideration. A parent as well as a nurse or physician should accompany the infant with relevant information and x-rays.

Infants with serious respiratory or circulatory disturbances are best transported after resuscitation has been started and body functions are improving. An infant who has diaphragmatic hernia or intestinal obstruction should have a nasogastric tube passed into the stomach so that it can be emptied to avoid lethal aspiration in transit. This may also help alleviate respiratory distress. Suction apparatus should be available in the vehicle.

One of the best ways to prevent deterioration of an infant's condition is to use a portable incubator. Although an infant may be protected from excessive heat loss with warm wraps and hot water bottles, portable incubators maintained at 85 to 90° F are the most practical approach. Most of these devices have sufficient viewing room to allow for constant observation and care

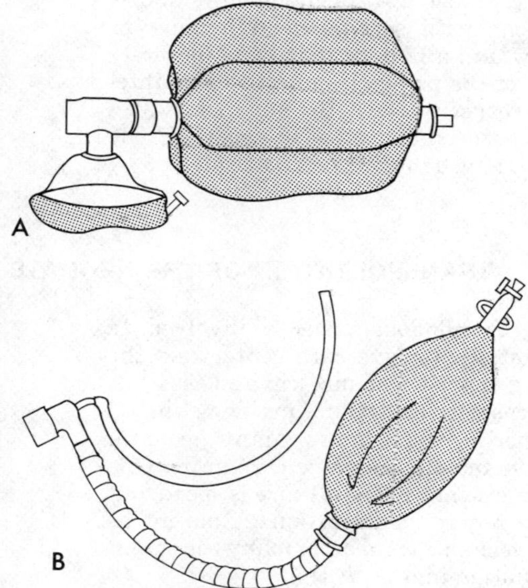

Figure 12–3 *A*, The infant Ambu bag. *B*, The Mapleson type ventilating apparatus.

of the infant while providing a warm environment. If assisted ventilation is required, it may be provided with an automatic ventilator or by hand using an Ambu infant bag or a Mapleson system (see Fig. 12–3). Care must be taken with the Mapleson system not to exert more than 20 or 30 cm of water pressure, whereas the Ambu bag is designed to limit pressure to a maximum of 40 cm of saline.

thermal, electrical, and chemical injuries

Tissue damage from thermal, electrical, and chemical energy will vary from insignificant to extensive, involving any or all organs and systems of the body. Early recognition of the seriousness of these injuries and prompt institution of appropriate therapy can reduce morbidity and mortality.

THERMAL INJURIES

Burns

The first consideration in caring for a burn victim is to stop the burning process. This may necessitate the removal of hot or burning clothing or hot objects such as belt buckles, straps, grease, tar, or other heat-retaining materials. The hands are the extremities usually involved in hot tar injuries (burns). To stop the burning process, a hand or foot can be placed in cold water for five minutes. This will cause the tar to harden and contract away from the skin, which will facilitate removal. The edge of a scalpel or hemostat can usually be placed beneath the hardened tar to lift it away from the skin. A portion of the epidermis or dermis will usually be removed with the tar, depending on the depth of the injury. After the tar is removed, the wound can be left exposed until the patient can be given definitive care. The hand should be elevated (on pillows) during transport, with active extension and flexion of the digits encouraged.

An evaluation of the patient should then be made to determine the seriousness of the injury. This should include the extent, depth, location, and cause of the injury and a consideration of the patient's age, preexisting complications, and associated injuries.

EXTENT. The extent of a burn is expressed as a percentage of the total body surface involved. A rapid method for evaluating the extent of a burn is the Rule of Nines, in which the body surface is divided into regions representing 9 per cent or multiples of 9 (Fig. 13–1). The extent of the burned area should be confirmed by estimating the extent of the unburned areas; the total should equal 100 per cent.

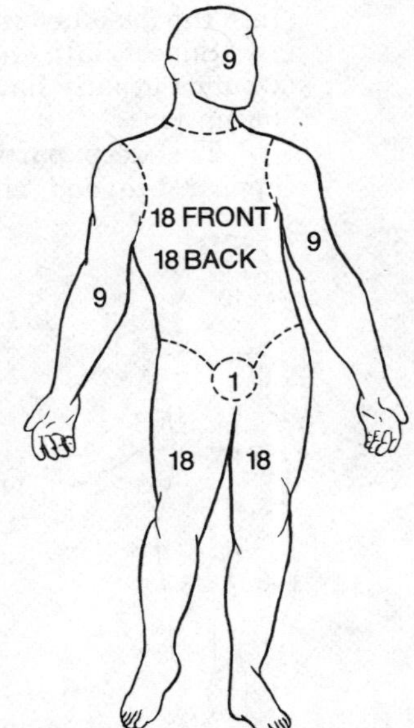

Figure 13–1 The Rule of Nines.

Children are an exception to the Rule of Nines. At birth, the head and neck area represents approximately 19 per cent of the total body surface, and the lower extremities represent approximately 13 per cent each (Fig. 13–2). For each year of age the head and neck area decreases by 1 per cent and each lower extremity increases by 0.5 per cent until age 10, when approximate adult proportions of the body surface are reached.

DEPTH. The depth of a thermal injury depends on several factors, the most important being the duration of the exposure and the intensity of the heat. Other factors are the anatomical location of the injury and the age of the patient.

Burn wounds are classified as either partial or full thickness. A *partial thickness* burn is an injury involving only part of the skin. A partial thickness burn may be further classified as *superficial* partial thickness (injuries involving the epidermis), *intermediate* partial thickness (injuries that extend into the mid-portion of the dermis), and *deep* partial thickness (injuries that extend into the deep layers of the dermis).

Superficial and intermediate partial thickness wounds usually have either a red appearance or blister formation.

The deep partial thickness injury has a marbly appearance and is difficult to differentiate from the

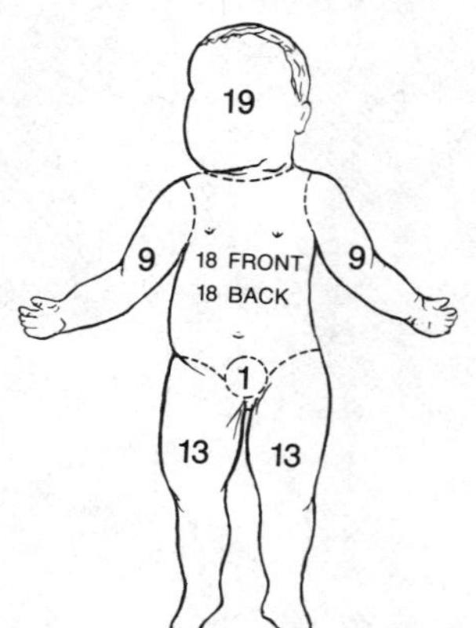

Figure 13–2 Diagram for estimating the extent of a burn injury in an infant.

superficial full thickness injury. An exact diagnosis of the deep partial or superficial full thickness injury is not critical, since the immediate treatment is the same.

The full thickness burn destroys all layers of the skin and, on occasion, involves muscle, bone, and other deep structures. Full thickness injuries can be identified by their charred appearance and a wound that is usually depressed from the surrounding area with visible thrombosed veins.

LOCATION. Burns of certain anatomical areas increase the seriousness of a thermal injury. When the injury occurs about the face and neck, the eyes should be carefully evaluated for ocular and lid damage. Edema may occur rapidly from burns about the mouth, nose, and oronasopharynx. Oral intake may not be possible, and intravenous fluid replacement will be necessary to maintain hydration. Occasionally, endotracheal intubation is necessary to maintain a patent airway.

Circumferential burns of the extremities may result in a constricting wound causing venous and lymphatic obstruction and, on occasion, decreased arterial blood flow. Circumferential burns of the trunk may restrict respiratory effort and may result in decreased oxygenation.

CAUSE. Certain types of burns have an increased potential for complications, thus increasing the seriousness of injury. When a burn injury about the face or neck occurs from a flame or flash and especially when it occurs in a closed area, the potential for a pulmonary thermal injury exists.

Flame or flash burns occurring in conjunction with an electrical injury demand a thorough evaluation regarding the electrical injury because electrical injuries are often more serious than burn wounds. When an electrical or pulmonary injury is suspected, the patient should be transferred to an appropriate treatment facility as rapidly as possible.

AGE OF THE PATIENT. Burns, like other forms of trauma, have an increased morbidity and mortality in infants and in the elderly. Therefore, smaller burn injuries in these age groups may require earlier and more vigorous fluid therapy. There is also a greater likelihood of fluid overload, renal failure, pulmonary edema, and electrolyte imbalance in burn patients in these age groups.

PREEXISTING DISEASE AND ASSOCIATED INJURY. Cardiac or renal disease and diabetes are examples of preexisting conditions that may increase the seriousness of a burn injury. Fluid replacement should be approached cautiously in the patient with cardiac or renal impairment, and wound management should be meticulously applied in the diabetic.

Other injuries concurrent with a burn can often be suspected from the history of the injury. Automobile, airplane, and other vehicular accidents frequently result in fractures and chest, abdominal, and head injuries. Each of these injuries should be suspected and appropriately treated.

Initial Care and Transportation

Following an evaluation of the extent, depth, and cause of injury and a consideration of the patient's age, preexisting disease, and associated injury, a decision can be made regarding the type of treatment required. If only outpatient care is required, the wound can be covered with a clean dressing during transport.

When hospitalization is required owing to the extent of the injury (20 per cent or more in adult cases, perhaps 10 per cent in pediatric cases) and a facility for definitive care is less than one hour away, the wounds should be covered with a clean sheet or dressing during transport. Situations requiring fluid therapy, endotracheal intubation, and splinting should be carefully evaluated prior to moving the patient and these measures appropriately instituted. Analgesics may not be necessary. Their administration can be deferred until a decision is made by emergency department physicians.

When the extent, depth, and location of the injury suggest that intensive care may be necessary, transport to an appropriate facility (not necessarily the closest) should be accomplished as rapidly as possible. In the case of serious injuries, the patient's condition will usually not improve or stabilize while awaiting transfer. If the definitive care facility is less than one hour away, intravenous lactated Ringer's solution should be started at a rate of 1000 ml per hour, and the wounds should be covered with a clean sheet or dressing. If the definitive care facility is more than one hour away, the wounds should be dressed with clean, but preferably sterile, dressings for comfort during transport. Analgesics (morphine, 2 to 4 mg intravenously) may be necessary in some patients but should not be given routinely. An exact record of all fluids and medications administered should be maintained.

Care of Associated Injuries

Most associated injuries take precedence over the care of a burn wound. Abdominal, chest, head, and extremity injuries should be thoroughly evaluated and treated before caring for the burn wound. Burn wounds can be cleansed with antibacterial soaps and detergents while other care is being rendered. Fluid replacement for thermal injuries will usually be a part of the therapy for serious associated injuries.

COLD INJURIES

Cold injuries can be classified as freezing and nonfreezing injuries. The freezing cold injury is commonly referred to as frostbite. The nonfreezing cold injury results from prolonged exposure to wet or moist conditions and is known as trench foot.

Mechanism of Cold Injury

The conditions that predispose one to a cold injury are low temperature and tissue exposure. Contributing factors include humidity or wetness, direct contact with cold objects, and lack of protection. The effect of humidity or wetness is readily seen when there is a hole in a glove or boot, allowing moisture to enter. Contact with cold objects, especially metal, will result in the rapid loss of heat. An exposed hand may often come in direct contact with a snowbank, a piece of glass, or other cold objects. A minimal amount of protective clothing is effective in preventing cold injuries.

The most important factor contributing to cold injury is wind velocity. As wind velocity increases, less time is required to produce a cold injury at a given temperature.

Treatment

Emergency treatment for patients with cold injuries is called for when there is cold or frozen tissue or when the patient is comatose or depressed. Coma in a patient with a cold injury is likely to be a result of prolonged exposure or alcohol intake.

Since patients with cold injuries are often hypovolemic, acidotic, and hypoxemic, intravenous fluids should be started if definitive medical care is more than one or two hours away. The comatose patient with a cold injury should be infused with a balanced salt solution (lactated Ringer's) containing 100 to 300 mEq of $NaHCO_3$, given at a rate of 250 ml per hour. Adjustments can be made after an arterial pH and peripheral hematocrit have been obtained and the urinary output has been observed for five or six hours.

It is preferable to obtain the arterial pH, pO_2, and hematocrit before therapy is instituted. If these determinations cannot be obtained before treatment and rapid rewarming of tissue is necessary, the fluid replacement rate should be increased to 500 ml per hour, because the rewarming is likely to increase the degree of acidosis.

To treat the hypoxemia that usually occurs in the comatose patient with a cold injury, oxygen should be given by mask or nasal catheter for six to eight hours or until the arterial pO_2 returns to normal.

Treatment of Cold or Frozen Tissue

A small number (1 to 3 per cent) of patients with cold injuries will present with cold or frozen tissue. If a definitive care facility is more than one or two hours away and the tissue can be kept warm, the cold or frozen tissue should be rapidly rewarmed. This is best accomplished by placing the patient in a tub of hot water. Normal adult skin will usually tolerate a water temperature of 100° F (38° C), and 15 to 20 minutes at this temperature will usually result in adequate rewarming of cold or frozen tissue. If rapid rewarming cannot be accomplished or if a definitive care facility is less than one hour away, the injured tissue should be covered with sheets or light blankets and the patient transported as rapidly as possible to the definitive care facility, with rewarming accomplished on arrival.

Most patients with cold injuries will not have sustained an injury severe enough to result in the freezing of tissues, and most will seek medical care after the tissues have been rewarmed. These patients rarely have emergent or even urgent problems. The damaged tissue should be protected from further injury and the patient transferred to a facility for definitive care.

ELECTRICAL INJURIES

The first priority in the care of a victim with an electrical injury is to remove the patient from the electrical source. This can be accomplished either by interrupting the circuit or by physical removal with a dry, nonconducting material such as wooden poles or boards.

Patients with electrical injuries should be transferred to an appropriate facility as expeditiously as possible, because tissue damage is commonly more extensive than it appears. Electrical current usually traverses several tissues from entry to exit, and the total damage is only partially evident from the skin involvement. Damage to muscle, tendons, nerves, vessels, and bone occurs frequently. If there is evidence of cardiac or respiratory arrest, **cardiopulmonary resuscitation** should be instituted.

p. 43

When the skin is damaged from an electrical injury, damage to deeper structures should be suspected. Tight muscle compartments should be decompressed and deep structures assessed for viability. With extensive tissue damage, fluid loss, acidosis, and myoglobinuria should be treated. When definitive medical care is more than one or two hours away, lactated Ringer's solution should be started intravenously at a rate of 500 ml per hour with 50 mg of sodium bicarbonate added until arterial pH can be determined. Close systemic and tissue monitoring is important in patients with extensive electrical injuries. Quality and quantity of the urine should be checked and recorded hourly. Arterial blood should be obtained every four to six hours for pH, pO_2, pCO_2, and hematocrit determinations. EKG monitoring should be continuous or at least frequent during the early phase of treatment.

CHEMICAL INJURIES

Prompt recognition and treatment of tissue injuries caused by chemicals may result in the salvaging of many organs and may reduce hospital stay and rehabilitation time.

Nature of Injury

Alkaline injuries are severely caustic. They result in deep and progressive injury to involved organs or structures. Acid injuries tend to cauterize the tissue, resulting in reduced available blood supply through thrombosis. Valuable time may be lost in searching for a solution to neutralize the chemical. Instead, the involved area should be bathed with a large volume of any liquid to dilute the effect of the chemical.

Specific Organ Injury

EYE. Chemical injuries are the most frequent cause of traumatic blindness. Acid injuries are seldom deep and rarely result in corneal damage. Alkalis, on the other hand, result in progressive damage to the cornea and frequently render the eye functionless. The severity of these chemical injuries can be significantly minimized by *continuous* and voluminous irrigation of the eye with water.

MOUTH AND PHARYNX. Chemical contact with the mucosa of the mouth and pharynx will result in a vascular response characterized by edema, subsequent thrombosis, and eventual scarring. The immediate management of these patients should include airway assessment, insertion of a nasogastric tube, and expeditious transport to a treatment facility.

psychiatric emergencies

The sudden and unexpected appearance of unpredictable or irrational behavior in a person is considered a psychiatric emergency. This patient requires immediate intervention to prevent harm to himself or to others around him.

GENERAL PRINCIPLES

The patient may be excited, agitated, restless, combative, quiet, withdrawn, or mute. What is most important is that his behavior is unusual *for him*. He may be disoriented (not aware of time or place), or his orientation may vary over time. On the other hand, he may be oriented but bewildered or confused.

The patient's thoughts may be disconnected, so that his speech makes little or no sense. He may talk very rapidly and may change from one idea to another with little or no logical connection between thoughts. He may even show evidence of auditory or visual hallucinations; he responds as if he hears or sees something that is not there. He may have fixed false beliefs (delusions).

The patient may be panicked to the point of speechlessness or screaming and may show aimless, meaningless movements of his body and limbs. He may also show the common indicators of intoxication such as slurred speech and ataxia.

The emotionally disturbed person may be frightened of his own feelings and what might happen if he does not control them. He may be frightened by the people and events around him because he perceives them in a distorted way and expects to be harmed. The violent physical activity of many but not all emotionally disturbed patients is generalized and is not directed against a specific person.

When initially encountering an emotionally disturbed person, take time to observe him. One member of the rescue team should be the leader, and everyone else must follow his directions without question. Talk to witnesses, friends, and relatives, and elicit their assistance in talking to the patient.

Attempt to talk the patient into coooperating. Maintain verbal and visual contact. Indicate that you know the patient is frightened and distressed and that you are going to see that he gets the help he needs. Be firm and truthful. Demonstrate by speech and behavior that you are in control of the situation.

PHYSICAL RESTRAINT OF THE COMBATIVE PATIENT

Be prepared for immediate action should the patient not respond to verbal requests. When physical restraints are required, be sure to have enough personnel available to hold the patient. The stretcher and any necessary restraints should be ready in advance. The basket stretcher is especially useful in transporting combative individuals (Fig. 14–1).

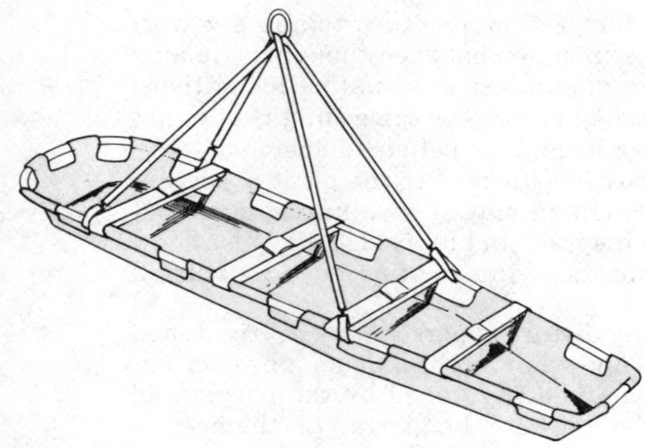

Figure 14–1 Basket stretcher.

ATTEMPTED OR THREATENED SUICIDE

Consideration of suicide is usually a response to chronic depression that has reached a crisis point. Suicidal patients remain oriented to time, place, and person but show changes in behavior such as slowed thought, speech, and movement or agitation.

The first thing to do is to engage the person in conversation. Recognize his despair and his difficulty in thinking clearly. Try to identify the problem and suggest possible answers. Suggesting the simplest and most obvious solutions may help the patient see some hope and may delay his carrying out the suicide attempt. Although the patient may sincerely intend to commit suicide, at the same time he may not really want to die. Once he agrees to accept help he will probably be cooperative, but be alert to any changes in his statements or behavior while he is being transported to the hospital.

TRANSPORTATION

Special consideration is required in transporting most emotionally disturbed persons because they will probably be awake and alert. They may refuse to be transported, and the assistance of police with their broader authority may be needed to hold someone against his will. Be familiar with state laws concerning taking someone to a hospital against his will. Often family and friends can convince the patient to go.

When transporting the patient, be sure he is secure. Keep the light level high in the ambulance to help maintain the patient's orientation. One attendant should stay in a position from which he can see and be seen by the patient at all times. Verbal reassurance should be continuous to maintain orientation and to lower anxiety.

If the patient refuses to be transported and his relatives will not or cannot convince him to go, they should be warned of the possible consequences, particularly in suicidal patients. Knowledge of your state's involuntary commitment laws will be helpful to families so that they can initiate appropriate proceedings.

MEDICATIONS

Antipsychotic Drugs

Haloperidol (Haldol) is a particularly useful tranquilizer in psychiatric emergencies because it is relatively nonsedating, it has little or no cardiovascular effect, and it is available in parenteral, liquid, and tablet forms. The usual dosage of haloperidol is 5 to 10 mg intramuscularly every 30 minutes.

Antianxiety Drugs

Diazepam (Valium) has antianxiety, anticonvulsant, and muscle relaxant effects, making it useful in psychiatric emergencies. It is available in parenteral and tablet forms. The usual dosage is 5 to 10 mg intravenously over two minutes every 30 to 60 minutes or 10 mg orally every hour until the patient is controlled.

administration of medications

An important feature of advanced life support is the early administration of medication. Of course, only certified paramedics are legally permitted to give injections, but drug therapy can also be administered by oral or rectal routes, both of which are practicable for the less-advanced EMT.

Before a medication can be administered, it must be identified by name and concentration. After this has been checked, the dosage must be accurately computed. Medications are commonly ordered in milligrams and milliliters, but some are still marketed in the apothecary forms of grains, minims, and ounces. If conversion from one system to another is required, use the following conversion factors:

```
grains  = grams × 15
minims = milliliters × 15
 drams  = grams or milliliters ÷ 4
ounces  = grams or milliliters ÷ 30
grams or milliliters = grains or minims ÷ 15
grams or milliliters = drams × 4
grams or milliliters = ounces × 30
```

Sometimes it is necessary to prepare a parenteral dosage from a hypodermic tablet, which is dissolved and injected. If the size of the hypodermic tablet is different from the dosage ordered but in the same denomination, use the following formula:

$$\frac{\text{dosage ordered}}{\text{dosage on hand (tablet size)}} \times \text{diluent/tablet} = \text{correct dosage}$$

ORAL AND SUBLINGUAL MEDICATIONS

Oral administration of medication should be utilized only in the alert patient who is capable of swallowing. If the medication is in a pill or capsule form, some liquid must be available to assist the individual in swallowing the medication. If the medication is in liquid form, some utensil for accurate measurement of the drug must be utilized.

Sublingual administration is the most common route for nitroglycerin, which is used in the early treatment of a patient suffering from heart disease with anginal pain. The medication, usually in tablet form, is placed under the tongue, and the patient is directed to hold it there until it is completely dissolved. Sublingual medication can also be in the form of a syrup that can be readily absorbed, such as a glucose syrup placed under the tongue of a diabetic patient in insulin shock.

RECTAL MEDICATIONS

The patient is prepared for rectal administration by being placed on his left side with his knees drawn up toward the chest. The medication, which is usually in suppository form, is then lubricated and placed in the rectum with a finger, which is protected by a finger cot or glove.

PARENTERAL MEDICATIONS

Parenteral medications are supplied in vials or ampules, which may be of unit-dose or multi-dose size. After computation of the dosage, the rubber stopper of the vial is cleansed with an antiseptic solution. An amount of air equal to the amount of medication desired is drawn up into the syringe prior to its insertion in the vial. This air is then injected into the vial to prevent a vacuum from being formed when the medication is drawn up into the syringe. The air will also prevent the loss of medication from the syringe back into the vial. After the needle is inserted into the rubber stopper, the vial is inverted so that the medication can be drawn into the syringe without air. The needle must be protected from contamination by preventing it from coming in contact with the edge of the vial during insertion and withdrawal.

Ampules are usually of unit-dose size. Since the ampule is made entirely of glass and has no rubber stopper, part of the medication solution usually is trapped in the neck and tip of the ampule. Gently shaking or tapping the top of the ampule will drain the solution back into the main body of the ampule. If the ampule is not prescored, the neck is scratched or scored with a file to ease the opening. With the fingers protected, quickly snap off the top of the ampule. To withdraw the medication, insert the needle into the neck of the ampule and draw the medication up into the syringe.

Prefilled syringes eliminate the necessity of withdrawing medication from an ampule or vial. The syringe must be identified by drug name and dosage. The correct dosage must then be computed if the syringe contains a different dosage. Since there are several different types of prefilled syringes, follow the directions closely in preparing the syringe. In the most common types, the barrel of the syringe is separate from the plunger, which contains the medication. Pop off the protective caps from both the barrel of the syringe and the plunger and screw the plunger into the barrel. Eject all the air out of the syringe before making the skin puncture.

Parenteral administration can be subcutaneous, intramuscular, or intravenous.

Subcutaneous Injections

A subcutaneous injection is made into the fatty layer of tissue just beneath the skin. Subcutaneous administration requires a syringe with a short, small needle (usually a 25-gauge, 5/8-in needle), a file if the medication comes in ampule form, and antiseptic wipes for preparation of the skin prior to injection. The most common sites for subcutaneous injection are the outer surface of the middle third of the upper arm, the anterior surface of the thigh, and the anterior surface of the abdomen. Prepare the site by cleansing it with an antiseptic solution such as alcohol or Betadine. Gently pinch the area between the forefinger and thumb so that the needle will go into the subcutaneous fat. After checking to see that all the air has been removed from the syringe, insert the needle to its full depth through the skin at a 45-degree angle with the bevel of the needle up. Release the skin so that the thumb and forefinger can stabilize the hub of the needle and therefore maintain the correct angle. Gently pull up on the plunger of the syringe. If blood is aspirated, withdraw the needle slightly before injecting the drug. If no blood is aspirated into the syringe, slowly but steadily inject the drug into the subcutaneous tissue. Quickly withdraw the needle and apply pressure over the site with an alcohol or Betadine sponge. Break the needle from its hub and the tip away from the body of the syringe and dispose of the needle and syringe.

Intramuscular Injections

Intramuscular injections are infrequently used in the pre-hospital phase of care. The syringe used for an intramuscular injection must have a needle long enough to inject the medication into the body of the muscle (usually a 22-gauge, 1½-in needle for an adult). A file (if the medication comes in ampule form) and antiseptic wipes for preparation of the injection site are also required. The middle third of the deltoid muscle is the most accessible site (Fig. 15–1*A*). The upper outer quadrant of the gluteus muscle can also be used (Fig. 15–1*B*). For ease of administration, the patient should be in the prone position with his toes pointed in. This relaxes the gluteus muscle so that the landmarks can be easily

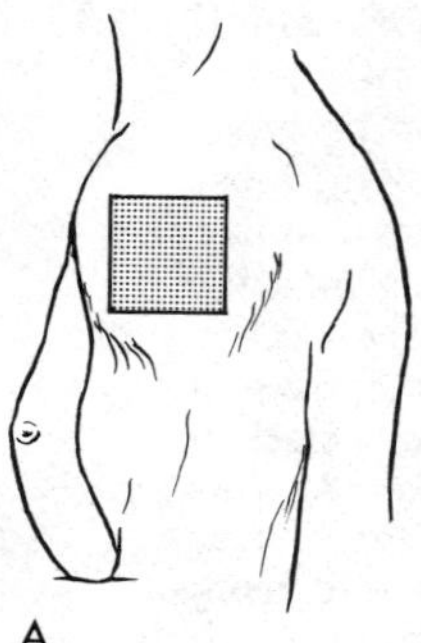

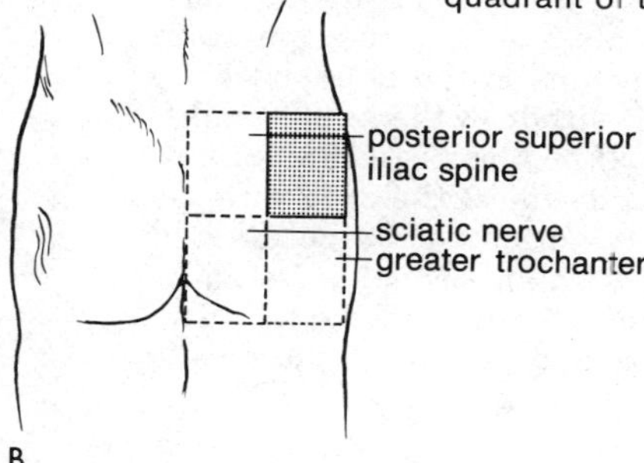

Figure 15–1 *A*, The middle third of the deltoid muscle. *B*, The upper outer quadrant of the gluteus.

identified. Draw an imaginary line from the greater trochanter of the femur to the posterior superior iliac spine. The injection must be given above and outside this line to avoid the sciatic nerve.

Another possible injection site is the vastus lateralis muscle. In the middle third of the thigh, this site extends from the mid-anterior to the mid-lateral thigh. A fourth site utilized for intramuscular injection is the ventrogluteal muscle. The patient may be lying on his back or side or he may be prone or standing. Place the palm of your hand on the greater trochanter of the femur and form a V by placing one finger on the anterior superior iliac spine and another finger pointing posteriorly along the iliac crest. The injection is made in the center of this V. The needle is directed slightly upward toward the iliac crest.

Prepare the site by cleansing it with an antiseptic solution. Remove any air from the syringe and stretch the skin over the injection site tightly with two fingers. Inject the needle through the skin at a 90-degree angle, usually for the full depth of the needle. Pull back on the plunger to determine whether the needle has inadvertently entered a blood vessel. If blood is seen in the syringe, withdraw the needle slightly until blood is no longer aspirated. If no blood is aspirated, secure the needle by grasping its hub, and steadily inject the medication into the muscle. Withdraw the needle and apply pressure over the injection site. Dispose of the equipment after the needle has been broken at the hub and tip.

It is important to insert the needle between the two fingers that are tightly holding the skin over the muscle so that the medication will not be forced from the injection site by a muscle springing back into its normal position (tracking).

Intravenous Fluids

Intravenous fluids are commonly classified as hypertonic, isotonic, or hypotonic (Table 15–1).

In the process of osmosis, fluid passes from an area of high concentration across a membrane to an area of low concentration. The relative concentration of solute to solvent (in this case, an IV solution and extracellular fluid) creates an osmotic pressure, or that pressure necessary to stop the flow of water across the membrane.

This osmotic pressure is measured in osmoles, the pressure (or number of particles) produced by 1 mole of solute in 1 liter of water. IV solutions are ordered in milliosmoles (1/1000 of an osmole). Plasma has an osmotic pressure of 300 to 310 milliosmoles per liter.

Table 15–1 CLASSIFICATION OF INTRAVENOUS FLUIDS

Type	Definition	Effect	Examples
Isotonic	*Same* number of solutes per unit volume as extracellular fluid	Will not affect water content of cells	D_5W (in bottle), lactated Ringer's solution, normal saline, blood
Hypertonic	*More* solutes per unit volume than extracellular fluid	Water will be drawn from cells	$D_{10}W$, $D_{50}W$, Plasmanate, albumin
Hypotonic	*Fewer* solutes per unit volume than extracellular fluid	IV fluid will pass into cells	D_5W, half-strength or quarter-strength saline in the body

Intravenous solutions can also be categorized as either crystalloid or colloid. A crystalloid solution, such as normal saline or lactated Ringer's, does not contain protein molecules. A colloid solution contains protein molecules, which, being large, cannot easily cross the semi-permeable cell membrane. Therefore, colloid solutions like albumin or Plasmanate have high osmotic pressures and are considered to be hypertonic.

IV fluids should be utilized in a patient suffering from trauma. If the traumatic incident has caused hypovolemic shock, the patient should be infused in the pre-hospital phase of care with intravenous fluids such as normal saline or lactated Ringer's, both of which are isotonic crystalloid solutions. Plasmanate is the preferred fluid because of its large protein molecules. The large molecules will draw fluid from the interstitial space into the vascular space and thus expand the blood volume.

In traumatic situations, the IV fluids should be infused at a rate consistent with the patient's condition. If the patient is in obvious hypovolemic shock, the fluid should be infused rapidly to stabilize the vital signs. If the victim has suffered severe head injuries, IV fluids should not be rapidly infused unless hypovolemia is also present. Head injury patients (if they are not in shock) are best managed with an IV infusion of isotonic crystalloids, such as normal saline or lactated Ringer's at a keep-open rate. Caution must be used when giving fluid therapy to the cardiac patient so that fluid overload does not occur. This means that the rate of the IV should be just fast enough to keep the IV line open.

Patients requiring maintenance IV fluid therapy are usually maintained on a crystalloid isotonic solution of normal saline or D_5W. Those patients on maintenance IV therapy that are also kept NPO are occasionally maintained on a hypotonic solution such as D_5W in half-strength.

IV fluids are normally not affected by wide ranges of temperature. IV fluids are usually stored at room temperature, which is 20 to 22° C. Each crystalloid IV fluid has a different freezing point, depending on its freezing-point depression. Cold fluids (temperature of below 5 to

10° C) should be used with caution in patients who are already in a hypovolemic state, since their rapid infusion may lower core temperature and further reduce the oxygen perfusion of the tissues.

Severely burned patients and patients suffering from cold exposure should have fluid administered at room temperature. If Mannitol is utilized in the pre-hospital phase, care must be taken to keep it at room temperature, since it will crystallize out at temperatures below 18 to 20° C. Crystalloid IV fluids are usually not affected by high temperatures. However, if Plasmanate is utilized in the pre-hospital phase, it should be kept at a room temperature of not over 30° C.

Equipment

When preparing for intravenous administration, the fluid to be utilized must be correctly identified and checked for clarity. The administration set must also be checked to assure that the fluid will be delivered at the proper flow rate and volume. If special filters are required, these must also be checked when assembling the IV equipment.

Standard IV administration sets usually divide each milliliter of the infusion solution into 10 to 15 drips. The mini-drip, or micro-drip, and pediatric administration sets deliver 60 smaller drips per milliliter. Some sets contain a small bag or cylinder at the proximal end of the IV bag that can limit the amount of fluid infused during a defined period of time. This is beneficial when a medication needs to be infused over a limited period of time.

Proper needles must be selected for the infusion of the IV fluid. Any needle, including those used in subcutaneous and intramuscular injections, can be utilized to perform the venipuncture. These needles are not used for continuous infusions, however, since they can easily penetrate the wall of the vessel and may allow the fluid to escape into the subcutaneous tissue.

Essentially, there are three types of needles or cannulas used for IV infusion. The butterfly needle is a hollow needle 1 to 1½ in long with plastic wings on either side to better stabilize the needle on the skin after venipuncture. A second type of intravenous cannula is the around-the-needle plastic catheter. The plastic catheter fits over a hollow needle. The venipuncture is made with the catheter over the needle. After proper placement in the vein, the hollow needle is withdrawn, leaving the plastic catheter in the vein. The plastic catheter is then attached to the administration set for infusion of fluids. A third type of intravenous cannula is the indwelling plastic catheter, which is inserted through a hollow needle. The danger with this cannula is that the needle can transect the plastic catheter, allowing a piece of the catheter to float free in the vascular system.

Tape must be used to stabilize the needle and administration set to the site of the venipuncture (Fig. 15–2). A nonallergenic-type tape is best.

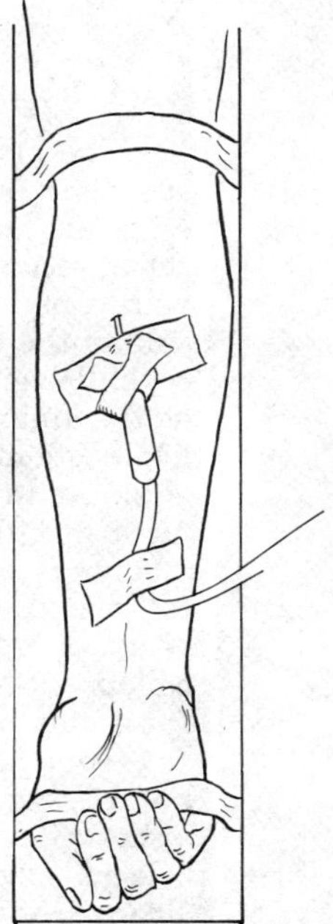

Figure 15–2 Securing an intravenous line.

A tourniquet is placed proximal to the site of the venipuncture. The tourniquet should be a flat piece of rubber, such as a Penrose drain, to avoid excessive pressure on the underlying structures. The tourniquet should be applied tightly enough to allow venous distention distal to the application without cutting off the arterial blood supply distal to the tourniquet.

Antiseptic swabs soaked in alcohol or Betadine should be utilized for cleansing the skin prior to venipuncture. In some emergency situations in the prehospital phase in which it is imperative that an IV be started immediately, asepsis is not always maintained. After the venipuncture, care should be taken to cleanse the skin thoroughly before the application of tape. When an indwelling catheter is inserted, the tape should be labeled with the date of the catheter insertion. Occasionally, an antibiotic ointment is applied to the venipuncture site to prevent local phlebitis.

Venipuncture

The most common venipuncture sites for intravenous therapy are the veins in the hands and arms, especially in the dorsa of the hands and wrists and at the antecubital fossae (Fig. 15–3). The superficial radial vein runs laterally up the forearm on the dorsal radial side to the antecubital fossa, where it joins the median cephalic vein to form the cephalic vein. Superficial veins on the ulnar side of the forearm run up to the antecubital fossa to join the median basilic vein to form the basilic vein. At the antecubital fossa the median vein of the forearm bifurcates to become the median cephalic and median basilic veins. These veins are the most accessible for venipuncture. The distal veins of the arm should be selected first. However, if the patient is in circulatory collapse, the larger superficial veins in the antecubital fossa may be selected.

The procedure for venipuncture of the dorsum of the hand or forearm is the same as that of the antecubital area. After applying the tourniquet proximal to the selected site, the vein is located and the overlying skin is cleansed with an antiseptic solution. The vein is held in

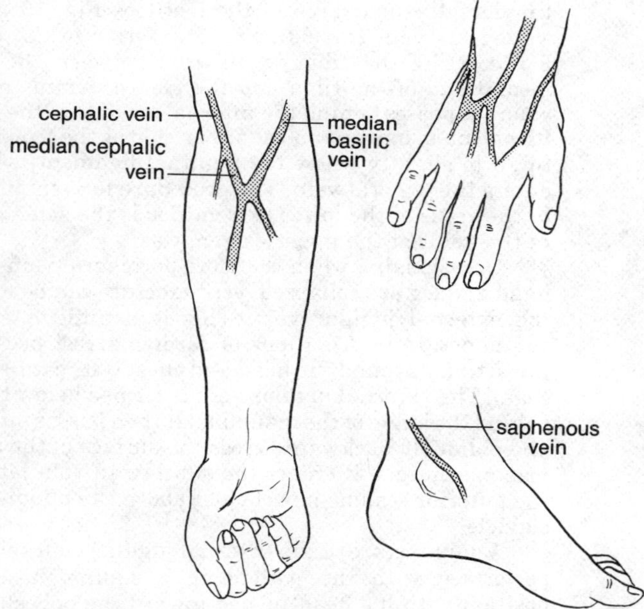

Figure 15–3 Common sites for intravenous therapy.

place by applying pressure distal to the point of entry. The venipuncture is made with the bevel of the needle up about ½ to 1 cm from the vein. The vein may be entered either from the side or directly from above.

When blood freely returns in the needle, advance the needle or the catheter into the lumen of the vein. If an around-the-needle catheter device is used, withdraw and remove the needle and attach the intravenous tubing. Secure the hub of the needle to the intravenous infusion site after connecting the intravenous tubing. The intravenous tubing is secured to the skin with adhesive tape. The hand and forearm may be anchored to an arm board (see Fig. 15–2).

Sites for intravenous fluid therapy in the lower extremities include the long saphenous vein, which runs on the inner side of the foot, receiving small veins from the dorsal venous arch of the foot (see Fig. 15–3). The saphenous vein travels upward anterior to the medial malleolus of the tibia to an area between the upper medial end of the tibia and the gastrocnemius muscle, where it passes behind the internal condyle of the femur. It continues upward on the inner side of the front of the thigh to slightly below the inguinal ligament, where it enters the femoral vein. The procedure for venipuncture in the veins of the lower extremities is the same as that in the veins of the upper extremities.

Occasionally, when the more peripheral veins of the hand and leg are collapsed, venipuncture can be made in the external jugular vein. This is a difficult site for venipuncture in situations of cardiac arrest because of the activity around the head and chest (i.e., cardiac massage). The external jugular vein is formed below the ear, behind the angle of the mandible. It then passes inferiorly and obliquely backward across the surface of the sterno-mastoid muscle. It enters the subclavian vein lateral to the anterior scalene muscle just above the middle of the clavicle.

Venipuncture of the external jugular vein should be performed with the patient in a supine, head-down position with his head turned toward the opposite side, which will allow for distention of the external jugular vein. After cleansing the skin, the cannula must be placed in the same direction as the vein, with the point aimed toward the shoulder on the same side as the venipuncture. The venipuncture should be made midway between the angle of the jaw and the mid-clavicular line, with the vein compressed slightly with one finger above the clavicle.

The skin should be punctured with the bevel of the needle upward about ½ to 1 cm from the vein. The vein may be entered from the side or from above. When free blood is returned through the needle, the catheter should be advanced over the needle. The needle is then withdrawn and the intravenous tubing attached and stabilized to the neck with tape. Because of the movement of the patient's neck, only a plastic catheter device is used for this type of venipuncture.

When access to the central circulation is necessary,

frequent sites for venipuncture are the internal jugular vein and the subclavian vein. The internal jugular vein emerges from the base of the skull and runs laterally and posteriorly to the internal carotid artery. Near its termination, the internal jugular vein is lateral and slightly anterior to the common carotid artery. The upper third of the internal jugular vein runs medial to the sternomastoid muscle. The middle third of the internal jugular vein runs posterior to the sternomastoid muscle. The lower third of the internal jugular vein runs behind the anterior portion of the clavicular head of the sternomastoid muscle and joins the subclavian vein just above the medial end of the clavicle.

The subclavian vein begins as a continuation of the axillary vein at the border of the first rib and then crosses over the first rib and passes anteriorly to the anterior scalene muscle. The scalene muscle separates the subclavian vein from the subclavian artery, which runs behind the anterior scalene muscle. The subclavian vein joins with the internal jugular vein to form the brachiocephalic vein.

A long around-the-needle catheter, usually 15 to 20 cm long, can be utilized for venipuncture of the subclavian vein. However, the through-the-needle catheter, which is usually a 14-gauge needle with a 16-gauge internal catheter approximately 15 to 20 cm long, is more commonly used for venipuncture of the internal jugular and subclavian veins.

The depth of the catheter should be determined by measuring from the point of venipuncture to the sternoclavicular joint, the mid-manubrial area, the manubrial-sternal junction, or approximately 5 cm below the manubrial-sternal junction. The tip of the catheter should be placed just above the right atrium for fluid administration.

Sterile gloves should be worn, and the skin around the venipuncture site should be prepped and draped as for a surgical procedure. The venipuncture site should be anesthetized with a local infiltration of lidocaine. The cannula should be mounted on a 10-ml syringe containing approximately 1 ml of saline or lidocaine. The patient should be placed in a supine, head-down position of at least 15° to allow for venous distention and to reduce the chance of air embolism. The patient's head should be extended and turned away from the side of venipuncture. It is helpful to place a roll of towel or bed sheet underneath the patient's spine between the shoulder blades to allow the shoulder to roll back and to allow easier access to the subclavian vein.

Place the fingertip of one hand in the suprasternal notch to establish a reference point and to locate the deep side of the superior angle of the clavicle. The course of the needle should be directed slightly behind the fingertip.

The needle is usually introduced approximately 1 cm below the junction of the medial and middle thirds of the clavicle. With the syringe and needle held parallel to the frontal plane, the needle is directed medially and slightly toward the head and should also be directed posterior to the clavicle toward the posterior superior angle of the sternal end of the clavicle.

The skin is punctured with the bevel of the needle upward, at which time the needle is flushed to remove any skin plug that may have occluded the bevel. After venipuncture, negative pressure should be maintained on the syringe as the needle is slowly advanced. As soon as the vein is entered, blood will appear in the syringe, and the needle should be advanced approximately 2 ml further to obtain a free flow of blood. Once the lumen of the vein has been entered, the bevel of the needle should be rotated caudally so the catheter can more easily enter the brachiocephalic vein. If the plunger of the syringe moves backward rapidly, this indicates that an artery has probably been entered. The needle should be removed and firm pressure applied to the venipuncture site for five minutes to prevent formation of a hematoma.

After the successful venipuncture, the syringe should be removed from the needle with the finger occluding the hub of the needle to prevent air from entering the needle and the vein. The catheter is then quickly inserted through the needle to the predetermined depth, and the needle is then removed from the skin with the catheter remaining in the vein. The catheter should never be pulled back through the needle, since the end of the needle could shear off the catheter, producing a catheter embolus.

The intravenous tubing is then attached to the needle or hub of the catheter, which is then secured to the skin with suture, making sure the lumen of the catheter is not compressed by the suture. The area is then dressed and the catheter taped in place.

Three approaches may be used to puncture the internal jugular vein. In the posterior approach, the needle is introduced under the sternomastoid muscle near the junction of the middle and lower thirds of the posterior border of the sternomastoid muscle. The needle is directed caudally and anteriorly toward the suprasternal notch at an angle of 45° to the sagittal and horizontal planes and with a 15° angulation forward to the frontal plane.

The internal jugular vein can also be entered by the central route. The needle is inserted in the center of the triangle formed by the two lower heads of the sternomastoid muscle and the clavicle. The needle is directed caudally and parallel to the sagittal plane. It is also directed at a 30-degree angle posterior to the frontal plane.

In utilizing the anterior approach into the internal jugular vein, the carotid artery is retracted medially from the anterior border of the sternomastoid muscle. The needle is introduced at the midpoint of this anterior border and is directed caudally toward the nipple on the same side as the venipuncture at a posterior angle of 30 to 45° to the frontal plane.

There are several disadvantages to using these central veins for venipuncture. The surrounding structures (the apical pleura, the lymphatic ducts, and the various nerves) can be damaged by persons inexperienced in the procedure. The venipuncture of central veins requires more training than does peripheral venipuncture. In a cardiac arrest situation, ventilation and chest compression have to be interrupted to cannulate these upper central veins. Hematoma and pneumothorax may be encountered with venipuncture of these central veins.

Another central vein that may be considered for

venipuncture is the femoral vein, which lies medial to the femoral artery immediately below the inguinal ligament. A line is drawn between the anterior superior iliac spine and the symphysis pubis. The femoral artery, which can usually be palpated, runs directly across the middle of this line. The femoral vein can be identified because it lies immediately medial to the pulsation of the femoral artery.

The preparation of the skin for the femoral approach is the same as that for the internal jugular approach. A 14- to 16-gauge around-the-needle catheter is commonly used. The venipuncture is made with the needle attached to a 10-ml syringe. The entry point is two fingers below the inguinal ligament medial to the artery, with the needle directed toward the head at a 45-degree angle to the frontal plane. The needle can also enter at a 90-degree angle until it will go no further. Maintaining suction on the syringe, the needle should be pulled back slowly until blood appears in the syringe, indicating that the vein has been entered. The syringe is then removed and the catheter inserted with the needle at an angle more parallel to the frontal plane.

The needle is then withdrawn, leaving the catheter in the lumen of the vein and the intravenous tubing connected. The hub of the catheter is secured to the skin with tape, and a sterile dressing is applied.

Occasionally, medications are added to the IV solution rather than administered directly to the patient. The drug and concentration should be properly identified and the correct dosage computed. The drug should be drawn up into a syringe if a prefilled syringe is not used. The rubber stopper on the IV bag is cleansed with an antiseptic swab and punctured with the needle, injecting the correct amount of medication into the bag. The needle is withdrawn, and the syringe and needle are disposed of. The IV bag should be immediately labeled with the name, dosage, and concentration of medication per milliliter of fluid in the bag. The rate of the IV fluid must then be calculated and checked so that the desired dose of medication is delivered.

If the medication is not to be added to the IV bag but is to be given directly into the IV tubing, the procedure is to identify the drug and compute the correct dosage. The medication is drawn up into a syringe, or a prefilled syringe may be utilized. The IV tubing is pinched off above the injection site of the rubber stopper. The rubber stopper on the IV tubing should be cleansed with an antiseptic swab before the needle is inserted. The desired amount of medication is then injected into the IV tubing, using the proper rate of administration for the medication. When the administration has been completed, the needle is withdrawn and the tubing unclamped to allow sufficient IV fluid to flow through the tubing and carry medication into the vein.

BIBLIOGRAPHY

Anthony, Catharine P., Kolthoff, Norma J.: Textbook of Anatomy and Physiology. C. V. Mosby, St. Louis, 1975.

Gray, Henry: Anatomy of the Human Body. Lea & Febiger, Philadelphia, 1973.

Hart, Laura K.: The Arithmetic of Dosages and Solutions. C. V. Mosby, St. Louis, 1973.

Intramuscular Injections. Wyeth Laboratories, Philadelphia, 1973.

Kaye, William Edward: Intravenous techniques. *In* A Manual for Instructor-Trainers and Instructors of Advanced Cardiac Life Support. American Heart Association, Dallas, 1975.

Tressil, Lawrence A., Grimes, Carl R., Gillelle, Joseph F.: Parenteral Drug Information Guide. American Society of Hospital Pharmacists, Washington, D.C., 1974.

Vanatta, John C., Fogelman, Morris J.: Moyer's Fluid Balance: A Clinical Manual. Second Edition. Year Book Medical Publishers, Chicago, 1976.

extrication and rescue

VEHICLE EXTRICATION

When accident victims are trapped in a vehicle, extrication and rescue proceed according to an organized plan designed to ensure prompt treatment. Elements of the plan include (1) support of an unstable vehicle, (2) gaining access, (3) initial assessment, (4) disentanglement, and (5) preparation and removal of the victim.

Vehicle Support

Extrication and rescue can be safely and adequately accomplished only after the vehicle has been supported and stabilized. To support an unstable vehicle, proper cribbing is needed, consisting of 2 × 4s and 4 × 4s measuring 18 in long. Each rescue vehicle should carry, as a minimum, 12 pieces of 2 × 4 cribbing and 10 pieces of 4 × 4 cribbing.

Cribbing must be placed where the structure of the vehicle is strongest and in such a manner as to prevent movement of the vehicle. If an automobile is on its side, best support can be obtained by placing the cribbing at the corners of the roof. Cribbing is also placed at the wheels. If the wheels are damaged or missing, support may be obtained by placing the cribbing at the corner of the rocker panel and the wheel well. If an automobile is on its roof, it can be stabilized by stacking cribbing from the ground to the hood and trunk near the bumpers.

Gaining Access

Try to open all doors first. If no doors will open, the next best means of access is to remove the windshield (Fig. 16–1). In the case of a windshield mounted in a grooved rubber seal, the rescuer need only run a linoleum knife between the glass and the rubber seal (Fig. 16–2). Inserting a bale hook between the windshield and the rubber seal forces the windshield out of the seal. In an older automobile, the glass will have adhered to the rubber seal and may crack while being removed. There

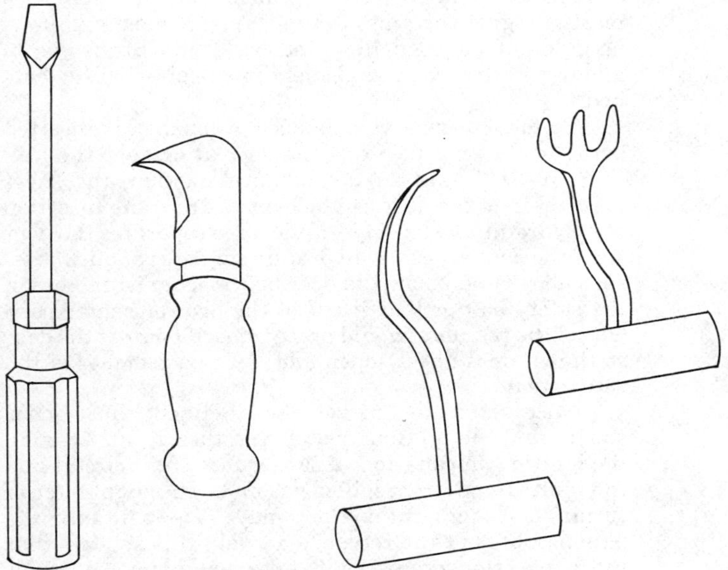

Figure 16–1 Tools required to remove a windshield.

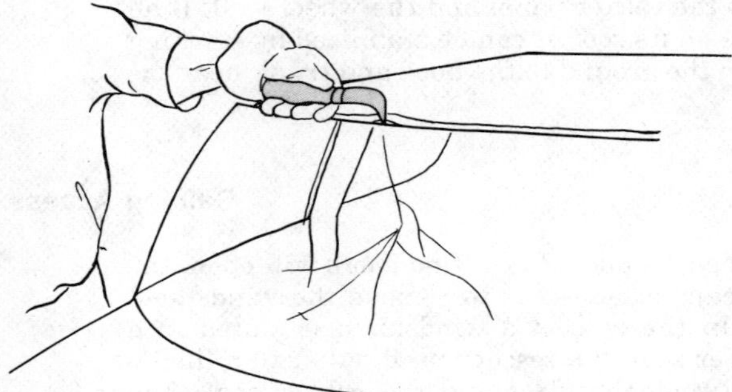

Figure 16–2 Separating windshield glass from its rubber seal with a tile knife.

will be some fragmentation and splintering of the glass, but the windshield will remain basically intact.

Newer vehicles have a windshield seal that uses mastic to glue the glass to the frame. A mastic knife is used to cut between the windshield and the frame to allow removal of the windshield in one piece with a bale hook.

To force open a vehicle door, a pry bar is inserted between the door post and the door at or near the lock (Fig. 16–3). Using an up-and-down motion, the sheet metal skin of the door can be bent to allow the insertion of a hydraulic wedge. Hydraulic force separates the door from the center post. A hydraulic spreader applies pressure above and below the door bolt mechanism to break the safety bolt or tear it out of the door or center post. One of the rescuers should brace himself against the door so that it does not fly open and injure a member of the rescue team.

Once access to the vehicle is gained, the rescuer should find the ignition switch and turn it off. Leaving the ignition on can cause a subsequent short circuit and can ignite fumes from spilled gasoline. The simple step of turning off an ignition key may save not only the patient's life but the rescuer's as well. If it appears that the extrication process will take some time, a better precaution is to disconnect the battery.

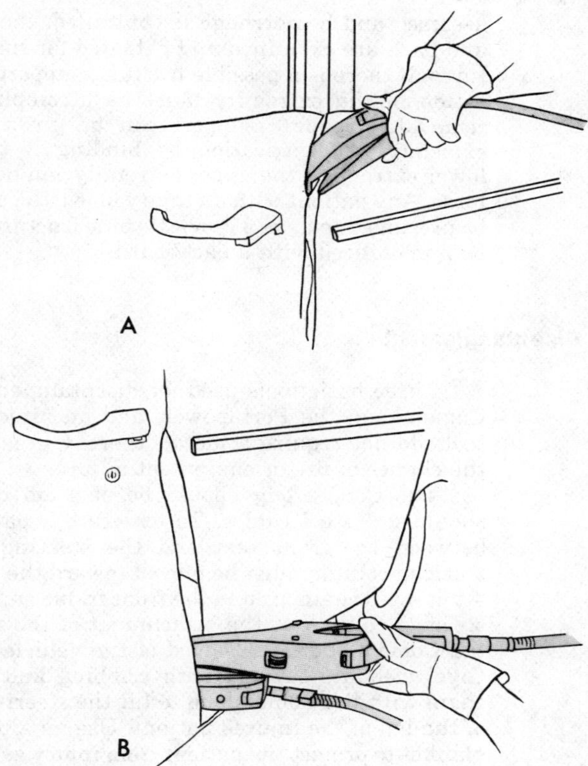

Figure 16–3 Steps in opening a door using powered wedges. *A*, Bend the metal skin of the door near the lock. *B*, Break the safety bolt by applying a hydraulic spreader.

Initial Assessment

An **immediate assessment** of the patient as to the extent of his injuries is made, and life support measures are started. After the airway and cardiac status are

p. 7

assessed and hemorrhage is controlled, the extremities and back are examined and palpated for suspected fractures. If there is a possible fracture, support and stabilization of the extremity must be accomplished before removal. Adequate support can be given to a lower extremity for extrication by binding it to the other lower extremity; the upper extremity can be fixed to the torso. Any patient with an injury above the clavicle must be presumed to have a cervical spine fracture and should be immobilized with a backboard.

Disentanglement

Three basic tools used for disentanglement are the Come-along, the Portapower, and an air chisel. These tools do not require a motor, thereby greatly reducing the chance of fire or equipment failure.

The *Come-along* should be of 4-ton capacity and should use steel cables. To extricate a patient pinned between the front seat and the steering wheel, the steering column must be moved toward the roof. Place a 4-ton rated chain around the front frame support and the steering column at the attachment of the wheel. Place the Come-along on the hood of the vehicle (Fig. 16–4). Give adequate support with cribbing and tighten the chain with the Come-along to lift the steering wheel out of the lap of the injured patient. Use an aluminized fire blanket to protect the patient from injury as well as from heat should a fire ensue.

A second common accident situation involves a patient wedged between the floorboards and the front seat. The seat must be moved while avoiding further injury to the victim. The Come-along is attached to the rear of the frame with a 4-ton rated chain. A second chain is placed around the seat. Steady rearward pressure is applied until the seat is suddenly jerked from its tracks. Protect the patient from possible rebound of the seat by placing a long spine board between him and the front seat. The Come-along can also pull a door completely around to the front of the vehicle, allowing easy straight-in access to the patient.

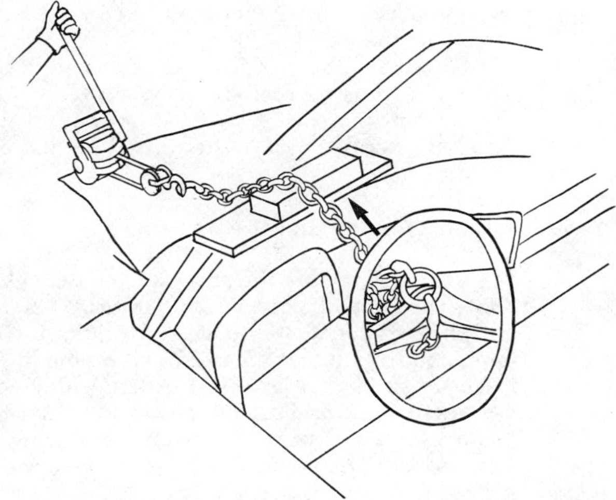

Figure 16–4 Moving the steering column with the Come-along.

The *Portapower,* with its various attachments, is also useful in disentanglement. The spreader or wedge can be used to straighten a floorboard bent around patient's foot, to break a seat loose from its tracks, to push a steering wheel out of the lap of an injured patient, or to move a dashboard. Additionally, the Portapower can be used to lift a vehicle to aid in freeing a patient trapped underneath.

The *air chisel* is the tool of choice for cutting into an automobile because it does not create large amounts of heat or sparks, which may cause a fire. Removing an injured patient from an automobile on its side by lifting him up through a door or taking him out through a window can further aggravate his injuries. An air chisel can be used to remove the roof in these situations. A three-sided cut is made from the lower rear corner of the roof, up and across the top, and down again to the lower front center. The sheet metal roof is folded down, and a tile knife is used to cut the head liner. If necessary, the roof supports are removed by cutting them with bolt cutters or the air chisel.

To remove the roof from an automobile that is right side up but has its roof structure flattened or damaged, cut through the corner posts at body level with the air chisel. The entire roof is then lifted up and off.

Preparation and Removal of the Patient

Before removing the patient from the vehicle, appropriate care must be given to his injuries (as found on the initial assessment). A suspected injury to the cervical spine requires an extrication collar and a short spine board for support (Fig. 16–5). A long spine board stabilizes the thoracic and lumbar spine (Fig. 16–6). Suspected fractures of the extremities require splinting. Accessible open wounds should be dressed to reduce the possibility of further contamination.

One person must always be in charge while the patient is being removed. This avoids further injury that

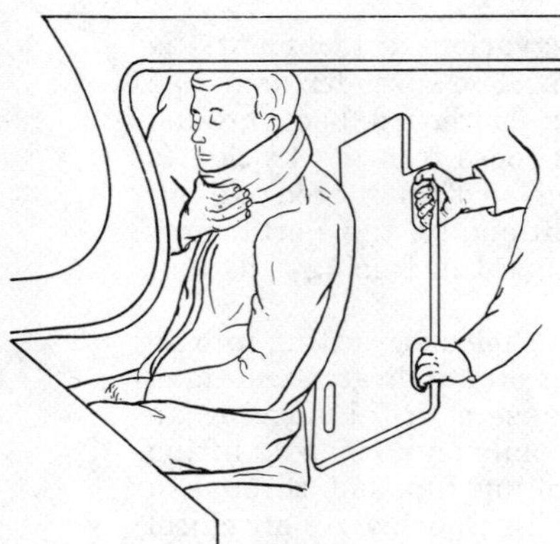

Figure 16–5 Placing the spine board in position before the patient is moved. A suspected injury to the cervical spine requires an extrication collar for support.

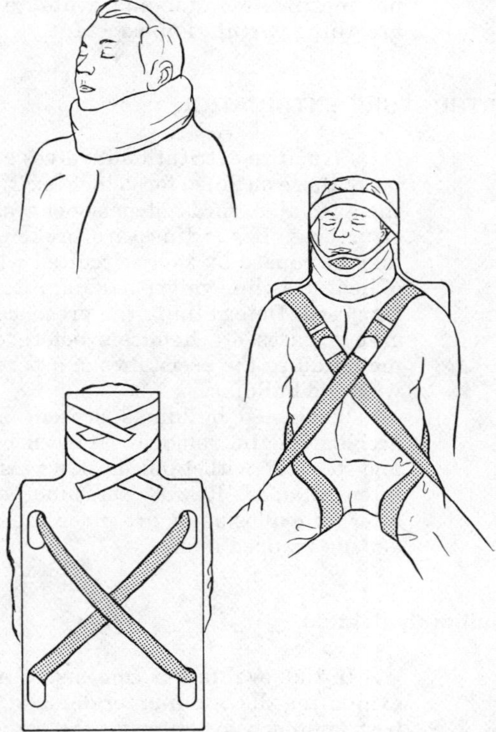

Figure 16–6 The patient strapped to the spine board for transportation.

may occur when one of the rescuers is not adequately prepared and the team does not work together as a unit.

Once the patient has been removed from the vehicle, a thorough secondary evaluation should be performed. Definitive measures that could not be carried out in the vehicle should be accomplished. These include full examination of the chest and abdominal cavities, further evaluation for suspected extremity fractures and head injuries, and treatment of associated soft tissue or internal injuries. Monitor and evaluate the ABCs (airway, breathing, circulation) constantly.

STRUCTURE EXTRICATION

Structure extrication involves a series of steps similar to those outlined for vehicle extrication in addition to the special hazards of poisonous gases and weakened structures. If gas lines are broken, explosion and fire may be caused by short-circuited wires or other sources of heat. Gas line valves leading into the building should be closed. Determining the presence of potentially dangerous gases or chemicals before entering a building may require the assistance of a person already familiar with the building.

Weakened buildings present a serious hazard to accident victim removal. Modern buildings of concrete and steel can withstand shock waves from explosions but later collapse. Rescue personnel entering a building after an explosion or fire place themselves in danger of getting trapped inside.

Initial Evaluation

Initial evaluation consists of assessing the scene, evaluating the building for damage, and deciding on the best approach for entering the structure. The information gained determines the course of action to be followed. When a potential for structural collapse exists, a decision must be made as to how and whether to attempt extrication of possible victims, giving consideration to the risk to the rescuers.

Gaining Access

Try the *doors* first. Guard against the potential hazards of fire or super-heated air by feeling the door. Do not open a door that has fire behind it. Self-contained breathing apparatus must be used when toxic fumes may be present.

If the door latch is jammed or locked, the next best method of approach is to use a pry bar. This method is useful only when the door and lock are of such construction that enough force to open the door can be delivered with a pry bar. Standard pry bars cannot break internal safety locks on many industrial buildings.

The power saw is another means of access through a door, even a steel door. The saw creates heat and sparks, and it should never be used unless fire protection is available with a charged hose.

Access through *windows* is quick and also allows a view of what to expect inside the building. The primary disadvantage is the time spent in dealing with broken glass. It is preferable not to break windows if they can be forced, pried, lifted up, or opened outward. This avoids the problem of crawling over, around, and through broken glass. The importance of wearing proper protective clothing when attempting any type of rescue cannot be overstressed.

Access through the *roof* can be accomplished through roof lights or roof vents or by using a power saw to cut through the roof structure. Two problems are encountered: first, the rescuer must walk on the roof, exposing himself to the dangers of a weakened structure. A life line is an additional and necessary piece of equipment in such a situation. The second problem is the threat of fire and toxic fumes when a roof light or exhaust vent is open. Making an opening in a roof may serve only to ventilate the building and may cause a smoldering fire to erupt into a rolling blaze. If toxic fumes are suspected, breathing apparatus must be worn.

If the stairs cannot be used, the easiest means of descent into a building from the roof is by rappelling. A properly designed rappelling rope, usually made of nylon, and either a fireman's rappelling belt or, if applicable, a Swiss-C made from standard braided rope is necessary. Dangers commonly encountered when rappelling are sharp edges cutting the rope and the possibility of lowering oneself onto a fire.

Gaining access from adjacent buildings can be accomplished through fire doors or by using a power saw to cut a hole in the wall.

Search and Locate

A systematic search plan is mandatory. If an organized approach is not used, the rescue team will be inefficient and may place their own lives in jeopardy. A working knowledge of the building and its interior is obtained either through a copy of the building plan or from someone familiar with the building. Determine the locations of doors, stairwells, and elevators, and particularly, information about any hazards that may exist. Even if it means briefly delaying the initial entry, every attempt should be made to obtain this information before the rescue plan is put into effect.

Initial Assessment

p. 7   Once the patient is located, an **initial assessment** determines his injuries and the care he will require. When structural hazards are present (e.g., threat of fire, potential for explosion, presence or suspicion of toxic fumes, the possibility of a weakened structure), the patient should be removed first and assessed later.

Disentanglement

Four basic tools can be used for removal of part of a structure that is pinning a patient. The Portapower and Come-along are used in structure extrication as in vehicle extrication. The chief advantage of the Come-along is that is uses steady, controlled power. The third tool is the air chisel, which is used to cut metal from structures. The fourth item is the power saw.

Preparation and Removal of the Patient

The principles used in preparation and removal of injured patients from vehicles also apply to injured patients in buildings.

SPECIAL RESCUE

Special rescue involves removing patients from remote or inaccessible places. Remoteness refers to distance and terrain as well as to obstructions such as snow, water, forest, or desert. Particular problems in special rescue concern access, identification and transportation of necessary equipment, and mechanisms of removal. Communication between the rescuers, medical facility, and the coordinating officer is a key factor. Special medical problems such as hypothermia may also complicate rescue.

Air Transportation

Helicopter

The vertical travel capabilities of the helicopter allow mountaintop or desert landings. The ability to hover permits a line to be dropped to hoist a patient into the helicopter from the water. The helicopter is also useful when available space will not permit even a vertical landing. The expense of operating a helicopter and its limited usefulness in ordinary rescue situations restrict its availability. Special rescue operations and hospital-to-hospital transfers are carried out by helicopter in areas where they are more common (i.e., mountainous regions) or when a Military Assistance to Safety and Traffic (MAST) unit is available.

The carrying capacity of a helicopter is limited by its width. A typical helicopter (in which two people sit side by side) cannot accommodate a litter.

Fixed-Wing Aircraft

Conventional airplanes generally are more available than helicopters but are less versatile in special rescue situations. Their size is more suited to carrying a litter and allowing continuous access to the patient. They can be operated at less expense than helicopters, and they can travel a greater distance in less time.

Land Transportation

Animals, particularly horses, are helpful on long treks across uninhabited areas, but provisions for them must be available, which generally means carrying food and sometimes water along. Although a significant amount of equipment can be carried by horse or mule, a patient cannot be transported successfully on a litter pulled by a horse or mule. Snowmobiles or dog sleds can be used for pulling a litter over snow.

A rough-terrain vehicle with four-wheel drive has many applications in special rescue if it is fitted with litters.

Communication

Communication between the rescuer and his base station, medical facility, or evacuation team is limited by the amount of radio equipment that can be carried into a remote location. A small transceiver that can be easily transported may have a communication capability of only a few miles.

Locating an accident victim in a remote region by radio decreases the search time; thus, it is desirable to have a type of automatic communication equipment that functions without fail. The Federal Aviation Administration has attempted to provide all aircraft with an impact-activated radio system, which transmits a carrier wave for location purposes, but the system is hampered by line-of-sight transmissibility.

The ideal solution in the future might involve a portable radio and a relay system via a communications satellite. In the meantime, a series of radio repeaters are helpful in regions where special rescue missions are frequent.

Equipment

Considerations of equipment for special rescue must balance usefulness against weight and size. A particular item may be absolutely necessary in a certain rescue situation, such as a special unit to deliver heated oxygen to a hypothermic patient or a spine board to a patient suspected of having incurred a back injury.

GENERAL RESCUE CONSIDERATIONS

Attention to the sequential steps of extrication and rescue will save the rescuer time and energy and will provide the injured patient with the quickest access to emergency medical care. As with any profession, the rescuer must be fully familiar with the tools available and must have a working knowledge of their advantages and disadvantages. Practice and more practice is the key to effective emergency rescue.

Of equal importance and concern to the rescue team is the proper cleaning and testing of the equipment after each rescue. Equipment that is overstressed or damaged during the emergency procedure will be discovered during cleanup and testing. If the rescue team does not take time to properly clean and inspect the equipment, it may well be responsible for increased danger in the next emergency when equipment fails at the scene.

Finally, the best training and equipment in the world will be of absolutely no value to the patient if the rescuer is not properly dressed. Persons involved in vehicle rescue cannot go to the accident scene in short-sleeved shirts or without gloves, goggles, or other protective clothing and expect to perform adequately. A qualified and competent rescuer may become another patient and an additional burden at the scene if not adequately dressed and prepared for the situation at hand.

index

Page numbers in *italics* refer to illustrations. Page numbers followed by a (t) refer to tables.